Walk Your Way Fit

Your Guide to Better Health, Wellness, and Vitality

Sarah Zahab

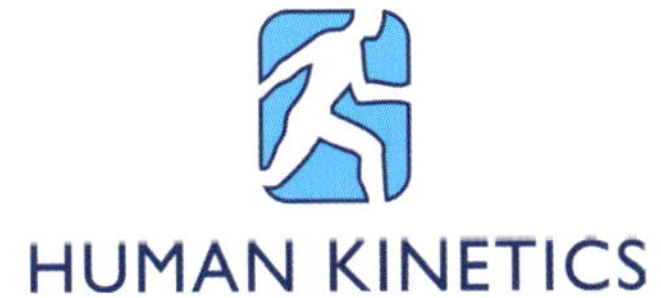

Library of Congress Cataloging-in-Publication Data

Names: Zahab, Sarah, 1977- author
Title: Walk your way fit : your guide to better health, wellness, and vitality / Sarah Zahab.
Other titles: Your guide to better health, wellness, and vitality
Description: Champaign, IL : Human Kinetics, [2026] | Includes bibliographical references.
Identifiers: LCCN 2025012915 (print) | LCCN 2025012916 (ebook) | ISBN 9781718236158 paperback | ISBN 9781718236165 epub | ISBN 9781718236172 pdf
Subjects: LCSH: Walking. | Walking--Health aspects. | BISAC: SPORTS & RECREATION / Walking | HEALTH & FITNESS / Exercise / General
Classification: LCC GV199.5 .Z35 2026 (print) | LCC GV199.5 (ebook) | DDC 613.7/176--dc23/eng/20250530
LC record available at https://lccn.loc.gov/2025012915
LC ebook record available at https://lccn.loc.gov/2025012916

ISBN: 978-1-7182-3615-8 (print)

Senior Acquisitions Editor: Michelle Earle; **Managing Editor and Permissions Manager:** Hannah Werner; **Graphic Designer:** Denise Lowry; **Cover Designer:** Keri Evans; **Cover Design Specialist:** Susan Rothermel Allen; **Photographs (cover and interior):** Gregg Henness / © Human Kinetics, unless otherwise noted; **Photo Asset Manager:** Laura Fitch; **Photo Production Specialist:** Amy M. Rose; **Photo Production Manager:** Jason Allen; **Senior Art Manager:** Kelly Hendren; **Illustrations:** © Human Kinetics; **Production:** Westchester Publishing Services; **Printer:** Versa Press

Human Kinetics books are available at special discounts for bulk purchase. Special editions or book excerpts can also be created to specification. For details, contact the Special Sales Manager at Human Kinetics.

Printed in the United States of America 10 9 8 7 6 5 4 3 2 1

The paper in this book is certified under a sustainable forestry program.

Human Kinetics
1607 N. Market Street
Champaign, IL 61820
USA

United States and International
Website: **US.HumanKinetics.com**
Email: info@hkusa.com
Phone: 1-800-747-4457

Canada
Website: **Canada.HumanKinetics.com**
Email: info@hkcanada.com

Human Kinetics' authorized representative for product safety in the EU is Mare Nostrum Group B.V., Mauritskade 21D, 1091 GC Amsterdam, The Netherlands.
Email: gpsr@mare-nostrum.co.uk

E9800

To John, Rayne, and Georgia:
You are my everything.

CONTENTS

FOREWORD

Running has been and always will be my greatest teacher. I've learned so much about myself and the world on expeditions and adventures spanning close to 20,000 kilometers. My path of adventure began as a way to change my life from a pack-a-day smoker, who was unhealthy physically and emotionally, to someone new. I never planned to be a professional adventurer—I just wanted to be happy. My brother John inspired me to step into the outdoors, and I never looked back. In my 30s, I became a passionate mountain bike racer. Then I discovered ultra running and completed ultras all over the world.

In 2007, my life changed forever when my buddies and I ran 7,500 kilometers across the entire Sahara Desert in 111 days, running on average 80 km per day. Soon after, we started my nonprofit organization, impossible2Possible, with the goal of giving young people an opportunity to be on expeditions and to learn cost-free. Since then, I have crossed almost every large desert on the planet in summer and completed many winter arctic Siberia expeditions. I trekked unsupported to the South Pole and attained the Guinness World Record for the fastest unsupported expedition in 2009. I'm a recipient of the Meritorious Service Cross of Canada, an Explorer in Residence of the Royal Canadian Geographical Society, Fellow of the Royal Geographical Society, and recognized by *Canadian Geographic* as one of Canada's Top Explorers. In 2024, I was awarded the Sir Christopher Ondaatje Medal for Exploration from the Canadian Geographical Society.

Twenty years of seemingly impossible adventures, expeditions, awards, educational opportunities, and traverses, yet much of that time was spent walking—most notably in my arctic expeditions, where running is not possible due to the gnarly terrain. Walking. Time on my feet putting one foot in front of the other, even when my body wanted me to stop. My motto is "limitations are 90 percent mental, and the other 10 percent is in your head."

Walking is one of the most basic forms of human movements. Through history, human beings transported themselves via walking. People crossed the Bering Strait and moved out of Africa on foot. Historically, walking has allowed us to survive. Most people can walk and gain with it a ton of benefits. Over my years of training, I've experienced numerous injuries, and walking has helped me complete the time on my feet required to do my best—one step at a time until the job is done.

Sarah has helped me keep my body healthy and happy for many years by correcting my muscle imbalances and helping me to run and walk injury-free. She's a wealth of knowledge, and this book will help beginning and advanced walkers alike. She guides people gently yet effectively. This book is perfect for anyone who walks, anyone who wants to walk faster, anyone who run/walks, and anyone who wants to gain a deeper understanding of walking for health and longevity. Sarah knows her stuff and walks the walk!

Ray Zahab

ACKNOWLEDGMENTS

This book would not have been possible without the help of many. I'd like to start by thanking Michelle and the team at Human Kinetics for your guidance. The entire team has provided incredible support, and I'm grateful for your hard work and assistance!

I'm so appreciative of all the contributors, who graciously shared words of wisdom and knowledge. Huge thanks to Roger Burrows, Ray Zahab, Dr. Kathy Dooley, Dr. Greg Wells, Joyce Shulman, Dr. Taryn Taylor, Jaime Sochasky Livingston, Jill Miller, Dr. Emily Splichal, Nancy Clark, Dr. Elizabeth Mansfield, Ryan Grant, Sylvie Gouin, and Malin Svensson. Your unique voices and expertise were critical in shaping this book.

A special thank-you to our wonderful models, Saleema, Colleen, Mike, Neil, and Michelle. You brought the pages to life!

An extra-special thank-you to Roger Burrows for being an incredible race walking coach and shaping my early race walking years. You've helped me fall in love with walking time and again. A big thank-you to the Ottawa Bytown Walkers and the club's coaches, Sandy and Joanne, for your ongoing support. Eileen, I'm grateful for your guidance.

I'm grateful for my team at Continuum Fitness and Movement Performance in Ottawa. Thank you for being the most incredible group of practitioners! And thank you to our amazing clients: Your support and encouragement have been so uplifting.

My friends have been integral in supporting me over the years. Leanne, Diane, and Aniseh: Love you to pieces.

I'm eternally grateful to my parents, who instilled a love of athleticism in me from a young age, drove me around from practice to practice and sport to sport, and supported me wholeheartedly. Miss you always, Dad. To my mom, Alsace: Your unwavering support means so much. You have been my champion cheerleader over the years, and your constant support has helped me in so many ways. Thanks, Mom! To Adam and Jadd, the best brothers out there: You're it!

Finally, I'd like to express my deepest gratitude for my husband, John, and my children, Rayne and Georgia. John: You are one of the most incredible humans I know, and I'm beyond fortunate to have you in my life. You are my pillar in all things—I love you. Rayne and Georgia: Words cannot express my deep and never-ending love for you. You are capable of amazing things, and I'm here to support you always and forever. I love you dearly—this book is dedicated to you.

CREDITS

Thank you to the following experts who provided information and quotes throughout the book:

Roger Burrows
Nancy Clark
Dr. Kathy Dooley
Sylvie Gouin
Ryan Grant
Dr. Elizabeth Mansfield
Jill Miller
Joyce Shulman
Jaime Sochasky Livingston
Dr. Emily Splichal
Malin Svensson
Dr. Taryn Taylor
Dr. Greg Wells
Ray Zahab

INTRODUCTION

Walking is one of the most basic yet underrated forms of movements. From birth, we roll, we creep, we may crawl, and then we take our first steps. The moment we're on our feet, a cascade of patterns, signals, activations, and feedback loops will shape our gait.

We walk for numerous reasons:

- to keep our hearts healthy, our bones and joints strong, and our bodies well
- to enjoy solitude, clear our heads, give our brains a boost, or garner new ideas
- to possibly find answers or forget
- to learn more about our environment, our communities, the people we know, and the natural world that surrounds us
- to provide exercise and fun for our beloved pets
- to spend time with friends and the people we love

We walk because most of us can. The handful of times I couldn't walk, because I was recovering either from injury or surgery, I could not wait to get back on my feet. Walking may be one of the most underappreciated forms of exercise, and perhaps it is only fully appreciated when we're unable to walk. And walking can be impactful and empowering. Walking is all-encompassing and uplifting: It enhances our overall physical and mental well-being.

This book explains walking from a physiological and biomechanical perspective. It covers aspects not only of fitness but also of overall wellness. We talk about how to walk well, walk faster, avoid injuries and modify if necessary, warm up and cool down properly, and walk in all types of environments and scenarios. Several walking workouts are included for all fitness levels to help guide you to walking your best walk.

The positive outcomes we can enjoy with walking extend beyond how our bodies look. Walking influences how we feel physically and how our minds operate and feel; it affects the interconnected aspects of health that go beyond calories burned. This book never mentions weight loss, calories burned, or body shape or size. This book is meant to be body positive and to focus on the numerous benefits walking provides beyond the scale. You'll find that walking provides infinite benefits—benefits beyond our aesthetic-based goals. Walking is for every body.

In easy-to-understand language, this book explains the anatomy and physiology behind walking, because the more we understand about how our bodies function, the easier it is to implement subtle changes when we walk. We'll elaborate on topics such as gear, terrain, and environment to help prepare and build up to that perfect step.

We'll review proper alignment and breathing, the foundation to set us up for success. We'll discuss gait mechanics, including what taking each step involves, from biomechanical, anatomical, physiological, and whole-body perspectives. Step-by-step.

This book covers walking from start to finish. It explains walking warm-ups—active and dynamic movements that will prepare all bodies for the most comfortable walk. Cool-down strategies and stretches are outlined with full illustrations and descriptions. You'll want to earmark those pages for that perfect, postwalk stretch.

Most important, we'll show you that you can walk fast, even faster than you thought, by highlighting amplification tips and strategies. Yes, walking counts as intense activity! We'll explain how to add intensity to your walks and make the most of each step.

Strength training is another key element to overall health and longevity, and walking alone is not enough. Loading our muscles, bones, and joints in a progressive way is important to help us reap the benefits of walking. Dozens of in-depth, fully detailed strength exercises are provided with colorful illustrations and comprehensive notes to help you get the most out of each exercise. Variations, safety tips, and modifications are provided for all fitness levels. We want to help you walk, and walk strong, for years to come.

Time-based and purpose-based plans are laid out for various fitness levels and goals. Do you want to work up to walking a 5K? Do you want to add some interval training to your walks? Are you new to walking and not sure where to start? The plans in this book cover each of those scenarios and more—all curated to help you walk comfortably, effectively, safely, and with strength and resilience, without having to worry about how many kilometers, miles, and minutes to add or change each week.

My goal is to inspire readers with more than just tips on how to walk, how to walk faster and farther, and how to walk for overall health. My goal is to inspire you to take those steps, take the extra steps, and take them regularly. That alone will allow you to reap the benefits that walking can provide. A consistent routine of walking, strength training, and varied activities allows our bodies to remain healthy, strong, and mobile for decades. To help, inspire, and guide you to walk your best, I am sharing proven tips and strategies based on my education, training, and experience as a Registered Kinesiologist, clinical exercise physiologist, former competitive race walker, and an avid walker who has led walking groups for decades.

Each page provides opportunities to learn more about what our incredible bodies can achieve, one step at a time. The what and the why, the how and the how-to, are outlined in clear detail, with full descriptions and images. This book is for anyone who enjoys walking, whether slowly or quickly, alone or with friends, short or long. It will help you to walk well, walk faster, walk safely, and walk injury-free for a lifetime.

Throughout time, we have walked. We have walked out of necessity, for pleasure, for fitness, for socializing, and for fun. With this book, you have a complete blueprint to help you enjoy and benefit from walking with confidence for years to come. Walk and be well. Now, let's take the first step!

PART I

FOUNDATIONS FOR YOUR TRAINING

CHAPTER 1

Benefits of Walking

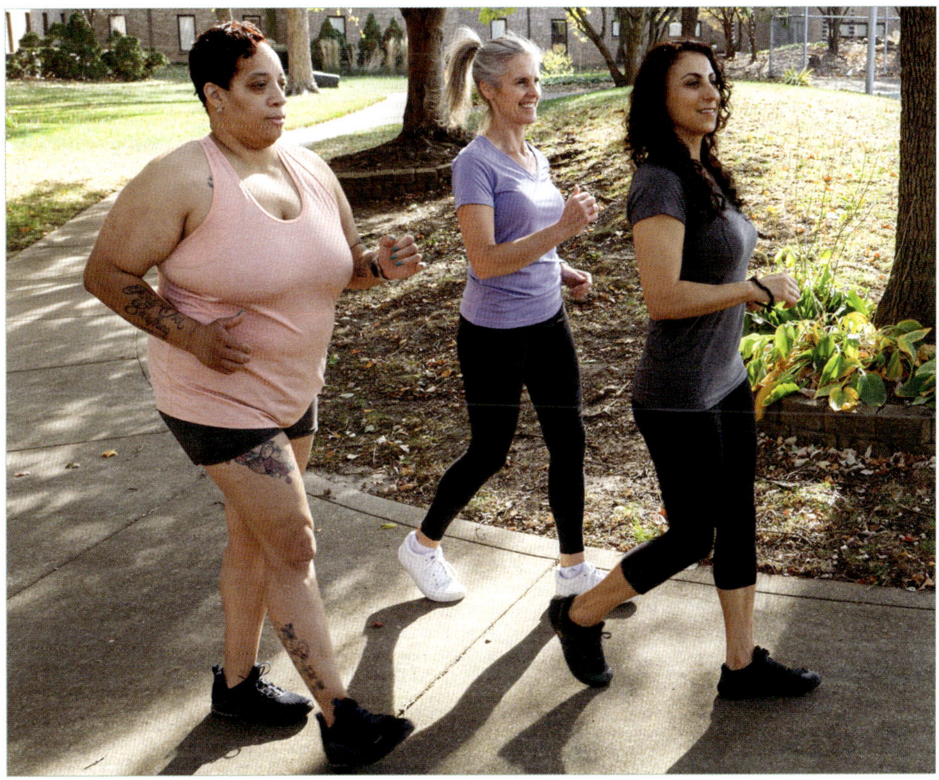

First we lift our heads. Then we roll, and we may creep or crawl. Finally, we walk. This may start at the age of one. Earlier for some, later for others. The time line doesn't really matter. We walk. We may not think about it, but we walk. We've been walking for millennia. We walk to get to places, we walk with friends, we walk for exercise, we walk our dogs—we walk for a multitude of reasons. We walk because we have to, we walk for joy, we walk to escape, and we walk toward the things we love.

The benefits of walking are numerous and proven. We can all agree that walking is a beneficial activity. Walking brings us so many valuable things. Even beyond the well-documented evidence and physiological benefits, there is immense, multidimensional value in the simple walk. Our hearts, brains, moods, and bones get a boost, but there's so much more to it. Joyce Shulman, cofounder of 99 Walks and author of *Why Walk? The Transformative Power of an Intentional Walking Practice* shares:

There is so much focus on the benefits of a regular walking practice for your body—which is fantastic. But often we overlook the powerful benefits walking delivers for your mind, your mood, and even your relationships. For many, it is those non-physiological benefits that are key to helping people stick to their walking routine because those benefits can show up immediately—from even one single walk—while many of the physical benefits can take weeks, months, or even years to become evident.

We're outlining some of the key benefits of walking to serve as a reminder, as a motivational boost, and as a reference, if needed. You likely don't need reminding, but just in case, let's try and inform you of the vast benefits of walking.

Disease Risk Reduction

Type 2 diabetes, Alzheimer's, dementia, cardiovascular disease, depression, obesity, cancer. Walking has been shown to be an effective tool to reduce the risk of these and other chronic diseases, including some types of cancer. A 2016 comparative study found that leisure-time physical activity, such as walking, was associated with lower risks of many cancer types (Moore et al. 2016). There were over one million participants in the study, and activities such as walking, running, and swimming reduced their risk of developing 13 different types of cancer. A 2021 study found that higher step count equated to lower risk of cardiovascular events and premature death (Sheng et al. 2021). A 2024 systematic review suggested that walking at faster speeds is correlated with a graded decrease in the risk of type 2 diabetes (Jayedi et al. 2024).

Granted, it's possible that many of the millions of participants in the various studies over the years have lower cancer risks because they engage in other healthy behaviors in addition to walking that may reduce their overall risk for cancer and other chronic diseases. Many of these studies adjusted for body mass index (BMI), smoking, and other factors; the evidence, however, surrounding walking as well as physical activity in general and disease risk reduction is robust and well documented. Walking is convenient, simple, and accessible. If we can live longer and more vibrantly while saving health care dollars in the long run, it's a worthy pursuit.

Injury Rehabilitation

Whether it's back pain, a knee injury, or recovery from surgery or various tendinopathies, walking can play a key role in bridging the gap from injury to a return to sport and life. Walking provides that time on our feet that allows us to continue grooving the linear pathways of ambulatory movement. It helps to reinforce the pattern of walking, hiking, jogging, running, rucking, and snowshoeing. As health practitioners who work with injured runners, walking is the primary modality to help improve overall threshold and tissue tolerance while we strengthen, address underlying issues, and allow sufficient tools and strategies for recovery. It buys us time while we rehabilitate, strengthen, stabilize, mobilize, realign, and make necessary corrections. Walking can be that first step to get individuals back to doing what they love. Walking was even found to improve neurologic function in individuals with spinal cord injury (Jones et al. 2014).

There are ways to work around multiple injuries and still be able to walk. With plantar fasciitis, for example, we can adjust our footwear, use different morning strategies when things are most uncomfortable, and prepare and warm up our feet, ankles, and fascia before walking. We may need to modify distance, intensity, volume, and time, but it can be done. Some is better than none. For some, water walking or water running can be great temporary options for those whose injuries prevent them from any load bearing activities. Many feel they must either do everything or nothing. Life is rarely black or white; so much exists in the gray. Don't be afraid to modify, tweak, adjust, or scale back temporarily if that is what you need to move forward in the long run.

Cardiovascular Health

Walking can be a moderate-intensity cardiovascular activity that helps to protect our hearts and reduces the risk of cardiovascular disease. Older adults who take more daily steps decrease their risk of cardiovascular disease (Paluch et al. 2023). The meta-analysis by Sheng et al. (2021) found that higher step count equated to lower risk of cardiovascular events and premature death, even with total step counts less than 10,000 steps per day. Another study found that brisk walking and vigorous exercise are associated with reduced coronary events among women (Manson et al. 1999). Walking is a good form of cardiovascular activity. Truthfully, although the studies are robust and contain large sample sizes, it is possible to obtain similar benefits from other activities. Many of the studies included individuals who were sedentary, and because of their inactivity, any exercise plan may possibly have created similar results. Although there are many forms of physical activity to choose from, walking is one of the most convenient, low-risk, comfortable, cost-effective, and simple forms of physical activity out there. For someone just beginning, it's an easy starting point to create a good foundation.

Walking can provide a good cardiovascular effort. I would argue that when walking briskly, with good technique and with power, it is possible to elevate your heart rate. When I was race walking competitively, I was able to get my heart rate in a higher zone and shift the pace from moderate to vigorous. Competing in a race walking competition was uncomfortable and challenging, similar to a running race. The pace of Olympic race walkers can average between 4 and 5 minutes per kilometer for a 20-kilometer race (faster speeds for shorter races). It's possible for Olympic race walkers to complete 5 kilometers in under 20 minutes. I don't know of many runners who can run that fast.

You don't need to be a competitive race walker to reap the benefits. But you can get a good cardiovascular workout when walking with the right technique. I run and I walk, among other cardiovascular and strength-building activities. I aim to run a few days a week and walk daily. Walking gives us that cardiovascular variety that is so important in overall balance. Mixing up your activities can boost your overall tolerance and threshold, prepare you for life's various demands, and build a resilient system. Performing a mix of low-, moderate-, and vigorous-intensity cardiovascular activities provides an overall balanced plan. Working in lower intensities helps build an aerobic base and foundation. Working in higher capacities helps boost overall cardiovascular ceiling and threshold. The moderate paces allow you to reap all the health benefits that walking has to offer.

Often, we discount walking, and many don't think of walking as an effective cardiovascular activity. There are ways to amplify, add power to, and intensify your walks. You'll find amplification tips and strategies in chapter 7.

Immune Boosting

In general, exercise boosts overall immunity. "Regular, moderate to vigorous physical activity is associated with reduced risk of community-acquired infectious diseases and infectious disease mortality, enhances the first line of defence of the immune system, and increases the potency of vaccination," according to a systematic review by Chastin et al. (2021). The lymphatic system, which essentially is part of our immune system, contains cells that help to ward off infection and diseases. Exercise, including walking, helps boost its overall function.

A study by Nieman (2011) with over 1,000 subjects found that those who walked 20 minutes or more per day for five or more days a week had 43 percent fewer sick days than those who exercised once a week or less. The subjects in this case experienced fewer upper respiratory tract infections overall, and the study was conducted over a fall/winter season when chances of contracting upper respiratory infections is usually higher, depending on where you live. Twenty daily minutes for fewer sick days seems like a pretty decent return on investment.

Even when sick with the common cold, Dr. Neiman, the author of this and other studies, recommends a brisk 30-minute walk if the symptoms are manageable and you feel like exercising. Sometimes that movement can bring us comfort, and it can be a realistic option if we're sick and unable to perform higher-intensity activities, if we can't congregate in indoor settings like gyms, or if we just need a little boost of fresh air and movement (Peachman 2022).

Brisk walking has been shown to improve endurance (Hardman et al. 1992). Ray Zahab, Canadian adventurer, founder of impossible2Possible, Royal Canadian Geographical Society Explorer-in-Residence, world record holder, author, and public speaker, shares his thoughts on the benefits of walking:

> At its baseline, people underestimate the effects of walking. Walking and running are biomechanically very different things, and they both offer different opportunities. Walking is a way of the body sustaining itself for extremely long periods of time. People have walked across continents. The movement of walking is probably the most human of activities (besides breathing, eating, and sleeping) that you can do. When you're exerting yourself at a very low intensity, you build without stress. Walking is a movement that you can do with very little increase in cortisol levels and instead a greater physiological adaptation, which means more capillarization by walking and breathing. The benefits of walking and running are distinct with some similarities: They are both cardiovascularly beneficial, but they are completely different in the way that the body adapts from the get-go and how basic a movement it is. Everyone can count their steps—it's the most accessible of outdoor and indoor activities that you can do.

Ray has been on numerous expeditions in some of the most inhospitable places in the world: the South Pole, the Sahara Desert from coast to coast, the Canadian Arctic, Death Valley (multiple times), and many other hot and cold deserts around the world.

> I run all the time for all my training, but walking as a mode of transportation for my expeditions is extremely critical; I spend 50 percent of the time walking because the terrain is harder. Just because you can run well doesn't mean you can walk well. Walking is very sport specific; you need to learn how to walk briskly and adapt to it. Walking is a tool in your toolbox. Sometimes I run, sometimes I ski, and sometimes I walk. Walking isn't a throwaway activity. To be really good at it, you have to practice it.

Steinhilber (2017), writing for NBC, labeled walking as the "most underrated form of exercise." Many different activities can improve our endurance, so it's important to find the one you can do consistently. For many, walking can be that activity, or the one that complements all the others, that allows you to build aerobic capacity to your fullest potential.

Mental Health

Although we may not have clear consensus on the exact amount required, a number of studies have linked physical activity with improved overall mental health (Hamer et al. 2008; Mahindru et al. 2023; Rodríguez-Romo et al. 2022; Singh et al. 2023; Bell et al. 2019; Chekroud et al. 2018; Stubbs et al. 2018). Teens who consistently participate in team sports in high school are less likely to be depressed as adults (Sabiston et al. 2016). We know that walking can improve your mood (Sakuragi and Sugiyama 2006).

Joyce Shulman shares her personal story of when she first discovered the power of walking at the age of 16. After arriving home from school in a terrible mood, her father, a lifelong athlete and coach who understood the power of physical activity, suggested she go for a walk before they talk.

> It was a beautiful spring day, and I walked two miles around my neighborhood . . . what I remember vividly, in one of those moments that you don't realize at the time will stay with you, was how my entire mood had shifted by the time I walked back in the door. It was at that moment that I realized that my actions had the power to impact my mood and that there are days when a single walk can change everything.

The Mayo Clinic (2023) tells us that exercise eases symptoms of depression and anxiety. Some studies go as far as to say that physical activity is just as effective as, or even more effective than, medication to treat mild to moderate depression (University of South Australia 2023). Hamer et al. (2008) found that a minimum of 20 minutes of any physical activity per week resulted in mental health benefits (walking was one of the activities in the study). Higher volumes and intensities correlated with greater risk reduction. Long-distance walking is positively related to mental health, according to a study by Mau et al. (2021).

I've been working with clients of all ages, from beginners to competitive athletes, for the last 25 years. Almost everyone leaves a movement session feeling happier, lighter, and sometimes high on that endorphin hit. I haven't yet come across anyone who regretted a workout. We rarely hear "I wish I didn't go for that walk." Next time you're contemplating going out for that walk, envision how you'll feel afterward. Often that's enough of a driver to get us out the door, even for short duration and distances.

Not a Cure-All

Despite the robust evidence showing the correlation between exercise and mental health, it may not be as simple as going for a walk. Yes, walking outdoors can be helpful and mood boosting, and in the long run, it's a great strategy to help improve overall mental health. However, after seeing a number of clients in the thick of depression (mild, moderate, or severe), it's not always that easy. Telling someone to "just go for a walk" or "just exercise, you'll feel better" may come across as insensitive. I opt to gently encourage movement—whatever movement feels best—and to support and celebrate any and all forms of activity. Sometimes and for some people, moving is just not possible. It feels too daunting, overwhelming, and not doable. The last thing we want is to add more stress and pressure. In my experience, giving that gentle nudge, acknowledging the difficulty of the situation, and encouraging all forms of treatment and strategies, including movement and outdoor walks, has been effective. It takes time, and respecting the process can be appreciated by those who may be suffering.

Brain Boosting

Walking has been proven to boost creative thinking (Oppezzo and Schwartz 2014). Another study found those who took more than 4,000 steps per day had healthier brain tissue in the area responsible for memory, learning, and cognitive function (Siddarth et al. 2018). Taking advantage of those postwalk boosts of creativity might be helpful in planning specific tasks. We often feel refreshed, invigorated, energized, and mentally sharp after walking or most forms of physical activity. If there's flexibility in your day, consider shifting certain work tasks to occur after walking. Or if you're finding it difficult to get through certain work or school projects, taking a short walk may give you a fresh outlook.

Our work culture has shifted over the years, and many of us spend long hours seated at workstations with fewer breaks. The return on investment in adding physical activity to your day is invaluable. Working longer doesn't always produce the same results. Working smarter by adding short movement breaks in your day can boost productivity. There is evidence that physical activity, even during work hours, boosts productivity (Coulson et al. 2008). Our overall work culture needs a shift to add in more incentives, opportunities, tools, and resources for employees to become more physically active. Some business leaders understand the power of walking and physical activity to drive creativity and innovation and have included parks (such as Apple Park) and on-site corporate wellness centers (Google, Apple, Microsoft). I first fell in love with power walking after seeing and eventually leading power walking classes in the corporate workspace. Employees went out for an instructor-led power walk in the middle of their day and always returned feeling better. I hope this trend toward more work–life balance continues, and opportunities to fit in more activity during our days at work and home increase. I hope the work culture continues to shift toward greater acceptance of physical activity as part of a healthy employee or leader.

Bone Building

Walking combines a low-impact effect with load bearing that helps increase bone density, especially in the trunk and hips, where many of us are screened and assessed. For postmenopausal women, who are at higher risks of osteopenia and osteoporosis, walking can be a great complementary activity to boost overall bone density. One 2022 study found that brisk walking for 30 minutes three times per week was an efficient way to improve bone mineral density (Lan and Feng 2022). The bone mineral density of the brisk walking group in the study was significantly higher than the sedentary group. Another study by Krall and Dawson-Hughes (1994) found that postmenopausal women who walked more than 7.5 miles per week (just over a mile a day) had higher bone density than women who walk less than 1 mile per week.

Strength training is without question a critical piece in increasing overall bone mass. Strength training is essential for everyone, especially as we age. Loading appropriately and working toward lifting progressively heavier loads is key. However, I have noticed in my 25 years of practice that my postmenopausal clients who consistently strength trained heavily three times per week were still seeing bone density declines with aging. These were women who were primarily cycling or swimming for cardiovascular activity, with some walking (or an occasional run). In recent years, I prescribed a more robust walking regime for my female clients in this demographic. In these women, after years of strength training, cycling, swimming, and occasional runs or walks, their bone density scores are improving with more time on their feet after seeing steady declines in various degrees. I don't have any scientific evidence to support this claim, because it's only what I have personally been seeing from a clinical perspective; yet the extra time on their feet via walking is potentially helping to boost overall bone density. For those who are postmenopausal or at risk of low bone density, osteopenia, or osteoporosis, strength training in addition to a regular walking program (or other similar load-bearing cardiovascular activities such as running) might be advantageous.

Social Connections

Being socially isolated is difficult for many. Walking with others adds a sense of social connection that's hard to quantify. Walking is a beneficial activity, and walking with others adds an extra layer of enhancement. Whether it is catching up with friends, hosting a walking meeting, participating in a walking group, or exploring the neighborhood with the family, there are many opportunities to increase social connections while walking. A *British Journal of Sports Medicine* study found that walking groups produce wide-ranging health benefits, both physiological and psychological (Hanson and Jones 2015). Joyce Shulman shares, "Walking provides one of the very best ways to connect with others. In fact, a survey of 2,300 women conducted by my company in 2019 revealed that while 73 percent of them acknowledged that they were sometimes or often lonely, those who regularly walked with friends were 2.5 times less likely to experience loneliness. What is it about walking together that is so powerful?" She believes the answer lies in the opportunities to remain present amid frequent distractions, synchronizing gait with others to build trust and affinity, boosting oxytocin levels (our feel-good hormone), and resolving conflicts by walking it out, the perfect tool to nurture relationships.

Many value the solitude of walking and believe the time alone allows for clear ideas to shine through, problems to be sorted out, and a sense of calm to take over. For those who are more social, meeting with or calling a friend or family member on a walk can be a classic two-for-the-price-of-one scenario. During the pandemic, for instance, we had to remain isolated to avoid spreading infection. Walking outdoors can be a viable option when indoor activities are limited and can allow us to remain connected with our friends, families, and communities.

Digestion and Hormone Balancing

We've all consumed large quantities of food at a holiday meal and experienced the sluggishness, discomfort, and fatigue kicking in. That walk after a meal can help! Walking after a meal has been shown to improve digestion, and it does not have to be long or intense to be effective. In one 2021 study, adults with a history of bloating walked for 10 to 15 minutes after each meal. After a month, they experience fewer gastrointestinal problems (Hosseini-Asl et al. 2021). Reynolds and Venn (2018) found that light exercise after a meal may reduce blood glucose levels, even just 10 minutes at a low intensity.

Walking was even found to help to regulate hormones—notably, those that help to prevent sarcopenia or muscle loss (Yamada et al. 2015).

Many of the studies used short periods of walking. Breaking your walks up throughout the day can be helpful, and saving a short amount of time for postmeal walking may give you that added bonus of improved digestion, blood sugar regulation, and hormonal balance.

Nature Therapy

Worldwide, people are spending less time outdoors. Adults and especially children are spending more time indoors. This phenomenon has been coined *nature deficit disorder*, and we're discovering that it's affecting our overall health and behaviors. Currently, no robust evidence backs up this view, but there are many conversations, articles, and spotlights worldwide regarding our exposure to nature and how it affects our development, behavior, mood, and even our immunity.

According to National Geographic (2019), forest bathing "emerged in Japan in the 1980s as a physiological and psychological exercise called *shinrin-yoku* ('forest bathing' or 'taking in the forest atmosphere')." The purpose was twofold: to offer an eco-antidote to tech-boom burnout and to inspire residents to reconnect with and protect the country's forests. This practice of ecotherapy has been shown to be beneficial and has been adapted by many countries and cultures. Forest bathing does not necessarily need to be performed in a dense forest to reap the benefits. Walking in any natural environment while consciously connecting to the natural elements around you is all it takes.

Grounding or earthing is another form of walking therapy that has been shown to be beneficial. It involves walking barefoot on natural surfaces such as grass, sand, soil, rocks, or concrete. According to Chevalier et al. (2012), grounding appears to improve sleep, normalize the day–night cortisol rhythm, reduce pain, reduce stress, shift the autonomic nervous system from sympathetic toward parasympathetic activation, increase heart rate variability, speed up wound healing, and reduce blood viscosity. Those walks on the beach are more powerful than you think!

White et al. (2019) reported that spending 120 minutes a week in nature is associated with good health and well-being. Spending time outdoors is invigorating, energizing, and mood boosting and gives us a dose of those feel-good hormones. Sunlight exposure in the right amounts can help us produce sufficient vitamin D levels, which are key for our health (depending on your climate). Exercising outdoors provides an exponential dose of all of those elements. This is especially true for those perfect-weather days when the temperature is just right and we're outdoors in one of our favorite places (a beloved trail; a tree-lined neighborhood;

a community garden in full bloom; a creek, river, or pond; or if you're lucky, the ocean), whether we're alone with the clarity to think about great ideas, answer tough questions, or ponder difficult situations, or whether we're with that person who makes our outdoor adventure that much more special. I prioritize tree-lined streets, trails, parks, and paths next to bodies of water. I live in Canada, and those perfect-weather days are mixed in with not-so-great days—really (really!) cold ones, icy ones, damp and drizzly ones, and very hot and humid ones. The temperature can go down to –40 degrees Fahrenheit (–40 °C) in the winter and up to 104 degrees Fahrenheit (40 °C) in the summer (not including the humidex). Going outdoors on those days can be a little trickier, but it can be worthwhile to make it work.

Investing in the right winter gear and footwear, finding alternate times to head out (e.g., early mornings or later in the evenings on very hot days), and prioritizing outdoor movement on nicer days are examples of how to make it work. We'll be providing tips on selecting the right gear in chapter 3. Of course, sometimes going outside is neither safe nor possible. Remembering how you feel after that outdoor brisk walk, jog or run, skate, hike, bike, ski, or other outdoor adventure can motivate you when you're contemplating heading out the door.

Cross Training

As someone who runs and walks, I find that walking helps to maintain a level of running fitness and economy when used in conjunction with a purposeful running plan. Depending on overall capacity, daily runs may not be possible for some. It may be difficult to recover fully before the next run. This is when walking on the off days can help to offer similar linear, ambulatory patterns, while loading in similar (lower impact) pathways. Time on your feet is key, and those miles (kilometers) spent walking can help build a robust system that's able to tolerate more loads.

Many runners will often use a 10:1 or 5:1 training and racing strategy—that is, 5 or 10 minutes spent running followed by 1 minute of walking. The minute spent walking can serve as a break and a chance to recover and actively rest. During race day, it can be helpful to keep a brisker walking pace to prevent a loss of race time (if there is a specific time goal). Some of the amplification tips and strategies in chapter 7 might help runners save precious seconds or minutes on race day. Keeping a speedy walking pace on race day walk breaks may help to shave time off total race time.

Convenience

Wake up, get dressed, put on shoes, head out the door. It can be that simple. Few activities are as convenient as walking. Depending on your environment and community, walking can be convenient, cost-effective, realistic, and easy to maintain long term for most individuals. When there are fewer layers of scheduling, organizing, and logistic details to sort out, we become more consistent with our walking regime. This consistency is what pays off in the long run.

In my years of experience, those who start small, progress slowly, and remain consistent are the ones who see the most results. Small steps done repeatedly produce great results. A 20-minute brisk walk may not seem like much; however, that brisk 20-minute walk done daily over a year will yield many returns. Don't discount the importance of small increments over time. It most definitely all adds up!

Longevity

Blue zones are areas around the world where people live longer. The highest concentration of centenarians (100 and over), nonagenarians (90 and over), and octogenarians (80 and over) live in blue zones. Currently, the blue zones are in Sardinia, Italy; Okinawa, Japan; Icaria, Greece; Nicoya Peninsula, Costa Rica; Loma Linda, California; and more recently, Singapore. People living in blue zones have similar lifestyle habits, such as having a sense of belonging, purpose, and positive mindset; eating well; and having a strong sense of community. They also move throughout their day, most of them walking as their primary form of physical activity. They may garden or hike, but most of them walk as part of their daily lives. They walk to the market, walk to church, walk with friends, and walk as a mode of transportation. Many of them live in terrain that is very hilly, providing a cardiovascular and muscular challenge to move around frequently in their daily lives.

A study of over 30 million people (Garcia et al. 2023) found that just 11 minutes of brisk walking per day (75 minutes weekly) can lower your risk of early death by almost 25 percent. Although many governmental organizations worldwide, including in Canada, the United States, and Europe, recommend 150 minutes of moderate to vigorous exercise per week, we're seeing that even a little bit can have positive impacts. The study has its flaws, as many do; however, the sheer amount of evidence linking physical activity and longevity is impressive. Some critics argue that the residents of many of the blue zones don't have accurate birth certificates and may be adding years to their actual age. I would argue that whether the adults in blue zones are 89, 91, 94, or 95, what they can accomplish is inspiring. They can squat (fully to the ground!), walk long distances, garden, and bend and move in ways that many North Americans at similar ages are not doing as vibrantly.

Studies have found that walking for longer periods of time, walking faster, and walking for longer distances are all associated with a decreased risk of mortality (Fujita et al. 2004; Dumurgier et al. 2009; Jayedi et al. 2022). Another study by Zaccardi et al. (2021) found that adults who walked at faster paces lived longer, irrelevant of BMI levels. Those who reported slower walking paces had shorter life expectancies. Inoue et al. (2023) also found decreased risk of all-cause and cardiovascular mortality in U.S. adults who walked over 8,000 steps, 2 to 3 days per week. Boosting longevity may not be the primary factor behind your motivation for walking, walking more, and walking with more amplitude, but who doesn't want to live longer and more vibrantly? I think many of us walk for different reasons—improving mental health, connecting with friends, getting from one place to another, or feeling good afterward—yet the overarching benefits can help to solidify our motivation for walking consistently.

Many forms of physical activity will help boost longevity, reduce disease risk, and provide many of the benefits listed here. If you run or do other forms of exercise at a moderate to vigorous pace, there's immense value in that. If you're sedentary or new to exercise, walking can be an easy, convenient, and doable form of activity to begin with. Complementing your cardiovascular activity with strength training provides a balanced fitness plan. You'll find more information on strength training in chapter 9.

Caveats

Although there are numerous benefits to walking, walking is not available and accessible to everyone. You may be injured or physically unable to walk. Not everyone has the physical capacity to walk, and this book isn't meant to be exclusionary to those individuals who are unable to walk. Certain environments make it challenging to walk outside. Very hot, cold, slippery, and icy conditions may prevent you from heading out the door.

In addition, living in a community where it may be unsafe to walk outside, alone or in groups, may make walking outdoors unrealistic. Safety is critical, and it may mean wearing reflective clothing and adding lights to increase visibility. It may mean avoiding walking outdoors altogether if you don't feel safe walking in your community. Not everyone has access to a vehicle to drive to a safer location or has time or funds to take public transit to a sports or public facility to walk indoors there.

Each situation is unique, and each individual must make decisions that are safest for them.

One block that is clear, safe, and usable might be your opportunity. Maybe it's around a government or public facility that is safer, kept clear of snow and ice, and more populated. You could perform repeat loops of one certain area as a backup option. While not ideal, it's an option for when paths, streets, and your specific environment is not usable.

Finally, you'll notice that we make no reference to fat loss, burning calories, or weight management as benefits of walking. Walking may have an impact on these elements; however, it was important for me to highlight the multitude of other benefits it offers. It is possible to walk too much. If you're walking for hours a day even when sore, walking excessively to burn calories (with or without restricting calories), or walking to maintain a low body weight, please seek help. This book is meant to be body positive and weight neutral; it's meant to encourage bodies of all sizes to walk in a way that feels right.

CHAPTER 2

Anatomy and Physiology of Walking

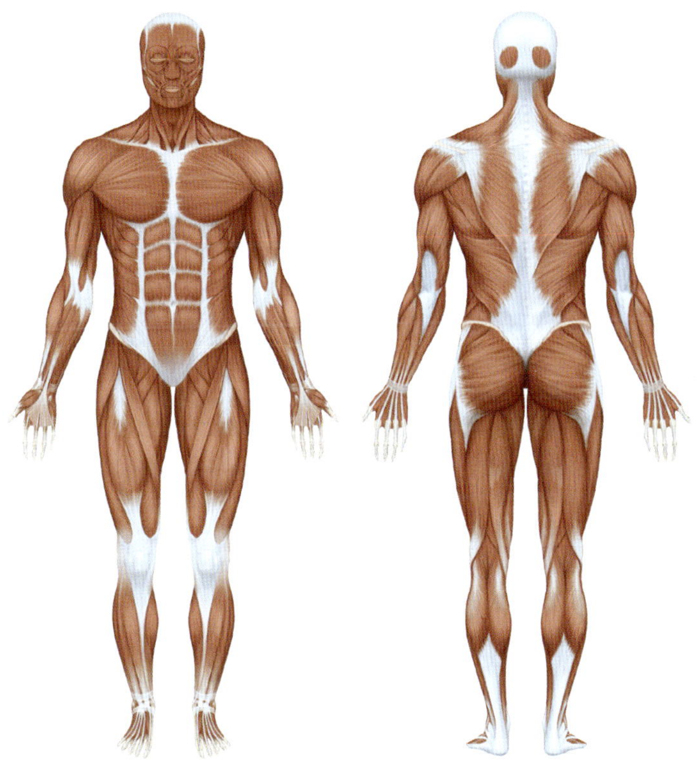

Of the roughly 600 muscles in the body, one could argue that almost all of them are used in some manner when walking. We're maintaining an upright position, having to use our postural stabilizers. We're moving in a linear fashion, having to propel ourselves forward using muscular forces. We're absorbing ground contact forces, striking the foot as we land and working up the chain to create accelerative drive. Our legs and arms have dynamic motion. Our back and core work to keep us secure and steady. When I first started power walking in my 20s, I was surprised at where I was feeling that postwalk stiffness and soreness the next day. I remember feeling the adductors, outer hips, and back muscles. It was enlightening. We will often feel that stiffness or soreness when trying new activities, working at higher intensities, or adapting to new movements. It's not a direct indication of how hard you've worked. It can be interesting (perhaps reassuring for some) to know that we've engaged a certain set of muscles.

Prime Movers

It would be difficult and maybe a touch overwhelming to describe here every muscle you use when walking. In this section, we'll explain the main prime movers and stabilizers being used in walking, as well as some key points on each (figure 2.1). Our prime movers are the muscles that are primarily working to produce movement. Although muscle has a specific role and function, we're ultimately looking at the integration of these muscles working as a whole to create clean, stable, functional, and effective patterns.

Gluteus Maximus

The gluteus maximus is the largest muscle in the body (figure 2.1*b*). It is your primary hip extensor—that is, it moves your leg behind you when walking. After landing, the leg moves under the body and behind you while remaining fairly straight. In a squat position, it helps to bring you up to a straightened position. In a bridge position on the floor, the glutes help to raise your hips.

In my years of practice, the glutes have been a topic of controversy. We should work on getting them to "fire." Some say they often "fall asleep" or "shut off." Others believe they should just work with larger global movements. I've come across many people with various injuries who have benefited from some sort of priming, correcting, or activation before loading. It's possible that the body creates compensatory patterns. Signals can switch, lines can get crossed, or connections can weaken due to several factors.

Typically, many strength coaches simply trust that glutes fire and train compound movements to load them. However, if someone is experiencing pain or discomfort, having a professional take a closer look (at the whole body) to determine whether anything can be done to correct movement patterns might be beneficial. If someone has been struggling with plantar fasciitis, I'll often check the glutes. Sometimes we see a connection between the calves, Achilles, and plantar fascia doing too much and the glutes doing too little. Similarly, hamstring strains or chronic tight hamstrings might result from the hamstrings doing too much and the glutes doing too little. This is what I've seen clinically in my years of practice. Preparing for movement with a dynamic warm-up provides a great opportunity to groove clean patterns and downregulate overworking

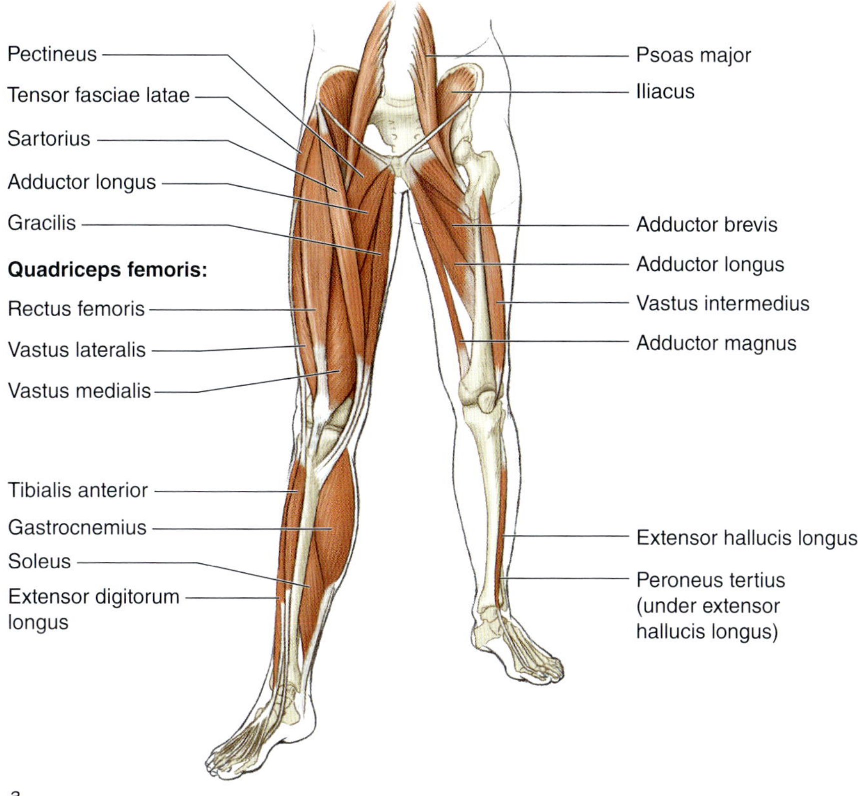

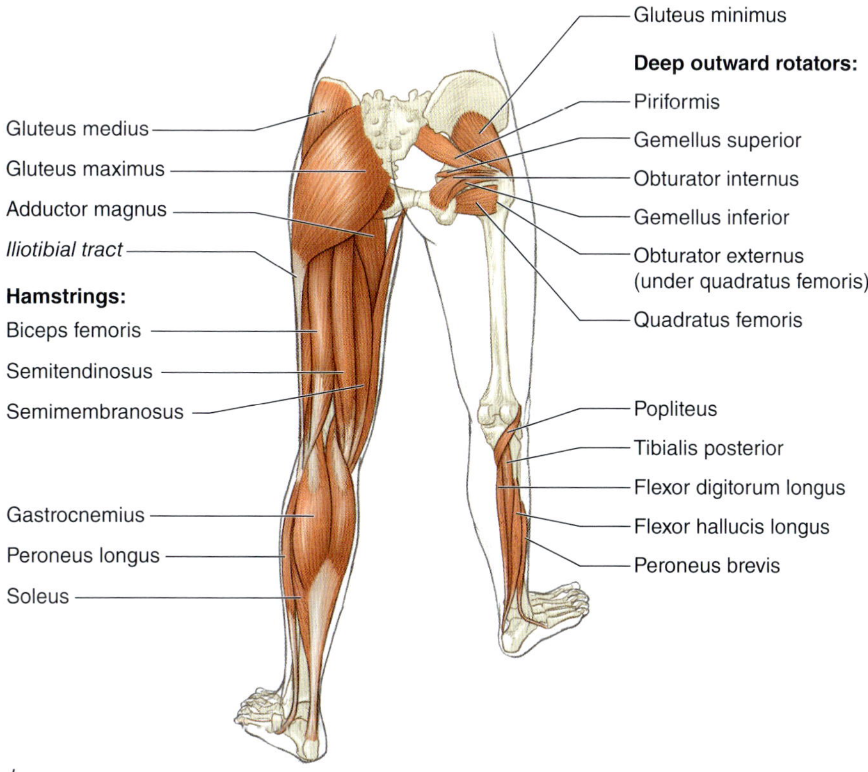

FIGURE 2.1 Muscles of the lower body: *(a)* anterior and *(b)* posterior.

areas while upregulating underworking areas. It's certainly possible to get up and go. However, taking the time to prepare, prime, and activate the body can lead to more comfort and ease during activities, especially as we age. It may be as simple as rolling or stretching the overworking area(s), followed by a few repetitions of a bridge or standing hip extension, being mindful to connect with the glutes before jumping into the desired activity.

Quadriceps

The four muscles that compose the quadriceps—the rectus femoris, vastus lateralis, vastus intermedius, and vastus medialis oblique—work to extend the knee or straighten it when the leg is bent (figure 2.1*a*). The rectus femoris flexes the hip. They all work together to stabilize the knee. When walking, the quadriceps straighten the knee as it comes through the swing phase before striking the heel down on the ground. This group of muscles is important to keep strong, not just for walking but for overall activities of daily living such as standing up from a seated position, sitting down from a standing position, or squatting down to pick up objects off the floor. In fact, studies have shown that those who have stronger quadriceps muscles have a decreased risk of all-cause mortality (Kamiya et al. 2015). Being able to independently get on and off seats, get dressed, and be mobile are critical as we age.

Hamstrings

The three muscles that compose the hamstrings—the biceps femoris, semimembranosus, and semitendinosus—are the primary knee flexors (figure 2.1*b*). They bend your knee back or bring your heel toward your hips. They also extend your hips and assist the glutes in hip extension. The hamstring group will fire after the leg hits the midline of the body when walking and moves the thigh behind you, and it bends the knee as you bring your foot off the floor.

The biceps femoris is the outermost muscle of the hamstring group and has two heads. The long head of the bicep femoris will extend the hip, flex the knee, and externally rotate the hip. This muscle will also rotate the lower leg out when the knee is slightly flexed. The short head of the biceps femoris will flex the knee and externally rotate the lower leg when the knee is slightly flexed. The semimembranosus and semitendinosus are the medial hamstring muscles. They are located toward the inside of the knee. Their primary role is hip extension, knee flexion, and internal knee rotation (turning the foot inward) when the knee is flexed.

You can feel the tendons of the hamstrings when seated by placing your hands behind your knee. Turn the foot inward and outward to feel the inner (semimembranosus and semitendinosus) or outer (biceps femoris) hamstrings activating.

Adductors

Five primary adductors adduct or bring the thigh in toward the body: the pectineus, adductor magnus, adductor longus, adductor brevis, and gracilis (figure 2.1*a*). They are key players in side-to-side movements. We don't adduct our legs a great deal in walking; however, they play an important stabilizing role, and some of the adductors have secondary roles.

The anterior fibers of the adductor magnus assist to flex the hip while the posterior fibers assist to extend the hip (with the glutes and hamstrings). The pectineus flexes the hip and also internally and externally rotates the thigh to some degree. The adductor longus and adductor brevis also flex the hip and assist in external rotation. The gracilis will flex the hip and act at the knee to extend and internally rotate the leg due to its lower attachments on the inside of the knee. We can't discount this important group of muscles, and training them helps to stabilize the pelvis and knees while walking. We'll cover some strengthening exercises for this muscle group in chapter 9.

Hip Flexors (Iliacus)

The hip flexors primarily comprise the psoas and iliacus (figure 2.1*a*). We sometimes see this group lumped into one muscle (iliopsoas). The two muscles are distinct and deserving of their own separate names. The iliacus is short and crosses one joint in the body. The psoas (addressed in the following section on stabilizers) has a different attachment point and crosses multiple joints. They will both flex your hip and bring the leg forward when walking. These muscles are often tight yet can also be weak. Stretching and strengthening them is ideally included in your overall fitness plan.

Latissimus Dorsi

This large muscle moves the arms and shoulders in various ways (figure 2.2). The latissimus dorsi extends the humerus (arm), pulls the arm into adduction (brings it closer to the body), internally rotates the shoulder (turns the shoulder inward), and even plays a role in assisting respiration as an accessory breathing muscle (more on breathing in chapter 4).

When walking, the lats pull the arm backward. The backward arm motion provides forward momentum when working to increase walking speed. These muscles are strong internal rotators (along with the chest

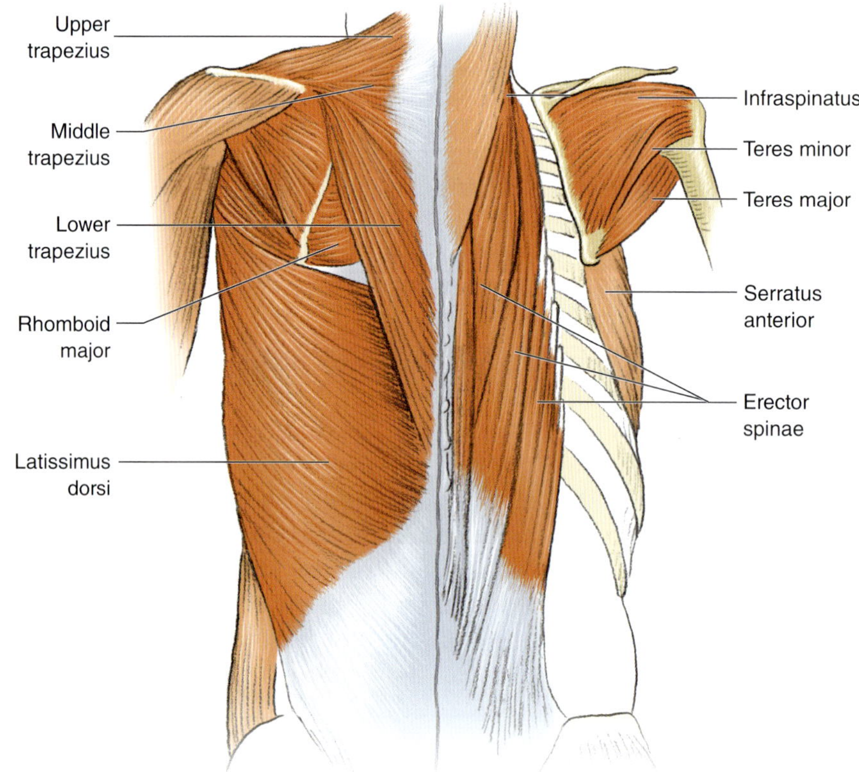

FIGURE 2.2 Muscles of the upper body: latissimus dorsi; upper, middle, and lower trapezius; serratus anterior; and rhomboid.

muscles), and ideally, we are working to improve balance in the shoulder area by including exercises that target the external rotators. This will help prevent a rounded, turned-in shoulder position and help create a more open chest/shoulder posture. We'll include specific strength training examples in chapter 9.

Posterior Deltoid

The posterior deltoid is a shoulder external rotator, horizonal abductor, and humeral extensor (figure 2.3). It will open the shoulder in (prevent the turned in hunched forward shoulder position) and extend the arm back and move the arm out to the side when it's positioned straight out in front of you (whether you are standing straight, leaning forward, side lying, or in an all-fours position).

This muscle is important when walking, because it helps to drive the arm back (humeral extension) while the opposite hip is extending in the

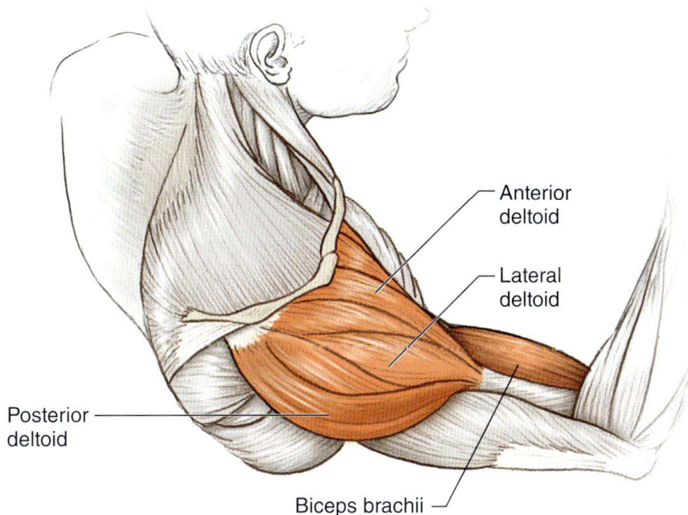

FIGURE 2.3 Muscles of the upper body: posterior deltoid, anterior deltoid, and biceps brachii.

toe push-off phase. This backward arm drive creates forward momentum. Punching the arms forward doesn't actually create forward speed. We'll be covering walking mechanics in more detail in chapter 5.

Biceps

The biceps brachii muscle flexes the arm (figure 2.3)—that is, it will bring your same-side hand to your shoulder. When walking, especially at faster speeds, our aim is to keep the arms flexed (think runner arms). This tighter position allows us to be more aerodynamic. A fully extended arm position will slow us down, and using the biceps to keep a tight, tucked arm position is ideal when walking briskly and looking to increase walking speeds overall.

Anterior Deltoid

This muscle is located in the front of the shoulder and flexes the arm forward (figure 2.3). When you reach for something, the anterior deltoid is helping to drive that movement. There are three parts to the deltoid: anterior, middle, and posterior. They all have different functions, and when walking, the anterior deltoid will swing the arm forward. Although we primarily focus on a backward arm drive, there is some forward movement, and the deltoids are working to hold the arm in a flexed position and bring it forward when the opposite leg is stepping forward.

Erector Spinae

This group of muscles runs the length of the spine and works to extend your back (figure 2.4). When working one side at a time (unilaterally), they will laterally flex the spine or bend it to the same side. They also help maintain upright posture and our natural curvatures of the spine. This is key when walking, because obtaining a stacked posture will minimize strain on other areas. Strengthening the back and building endurance safely to increase our tolerance works to potentially reduce back pain and expand our overall threshold and power output.

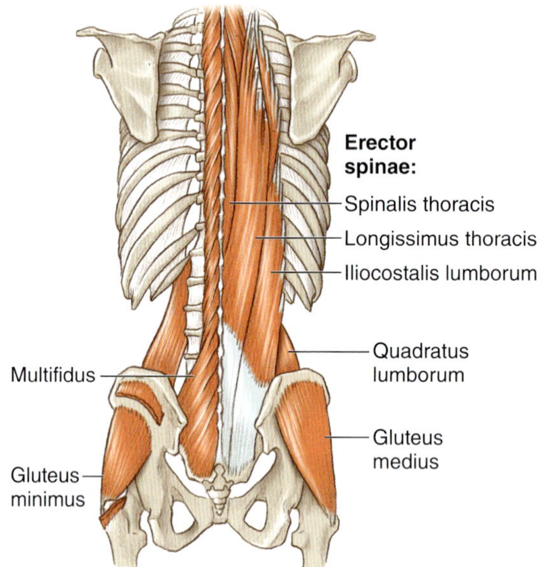

FIGURE 2.4 Muscles of the core: erector spinae and multifidus.

Calves (Gastrocnemius and Soleus)

Both the gastrocnemius and soleus work to plantar flex the ankle (point the toe) (figure 2.1). The gastrocnemius is more superficial, and the soleus is located deeper in the leg. This group of muscles is important in walking, because it pushes the ground away from us in the toe push-off phase. Ideally, we're pushing away from the hip and leading with the hip muscles, but some assistance with the calves may be beneficial in propelling us forward.

Tibialis Anterior

The tibialis anterior is our main ankle dorsiflexor (figure 2.1*a*). It lifts the toes upward when walking. This muscle becomes very important in people with Parkinson's disease and other neurological diseases. Lifting the toes quick enough to clear the ground is key to prevent tripping and falling. With my clients with Parkinson's, we work to strengthen this area so they can keep walking longer, more comfortably, and with fewer falls. Sometimes, a little extra focus on those areas can have a big impact.

Stabilizers

Our stabilizers are muscles that provide support, stability, and balance to keep our bodies moving well. They contract with other muscles to help hold us upright, and they respond to signals from the brain to modulate and manage pressures. As Charles Poliquin, Canadian strength coach, famously stated, "You can't fire a cannon from a canoe." We need stable surfaces to propel off of. If our foundation is wobbly, our output will be limited. Our small stabilizer muscles provide a secure foundation from which we can move freely, optimally, and powerfully. Figure 2.4 shows a few of the common stabilizer muscles.

Transversus Abdominis

Sitting deep in the intrinsic core musculature is the transversus abdominis (figure 2.5*a*). The fibers of this muscle run horizontally, like a belt. This muscle supports the thoracic and lumbo-pelvic regions, draws the contents of the abdominals inward, and increases intra-abdominal pressure. They work when you're exhaling forcefully, in conjunction with the pelvic floor, and as anticipatory muscles (i.e., they contract before your limbs do to support your spine and pelvis). Much of our power originates in the deep core, and ensuring we have good connection, coordination, stability, and strength through this region is important. You'll find core-specific exercises in chapter 9.

When walking, the core will fire to dynamically stabilize our back and pelvis. This action should ideally be reflexive. Holding the core tight all the time is not recommended when walking. Muscles need to relax and contract to fire optimally, and holding a gripped abdominal position at all times will affect breathing, the intra-abdominal pressure system, the pelvic floor, the back, and the pattern overall. We'll expand on breathing more in chapter 4.

Obliques

The internal and external obliques are your primary rotational muscles (figure 2.5*b*). Your internal oblique rotates you to the same side; for example, your right internal oblique rotates you to the right. Your external

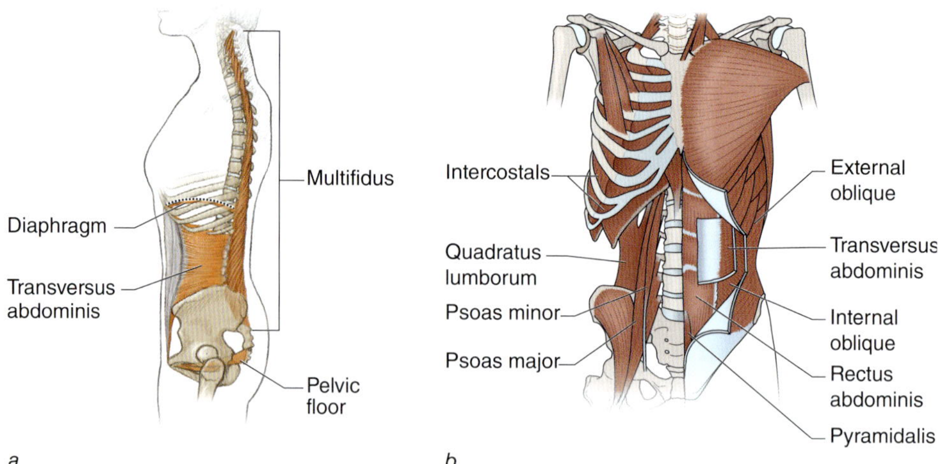

FIGURE 2.5 Muscles of the core: *(a)* transversus abdominis and *(b)* obliques.

obliques are opposite side rotators or contralateral rotators—for example, when your right external obliques rotate you to the left. Both internal and external obliques are same-side lateral flexors. Essentially, the right external and right internal obliques tip you down to the right side. They also play a role in stability, exhalation, compression of the abdominal cavity, and the left and right external obliques will flex your spine. The obliques also play an anti-rotation role. They stabilize your ribs and pelvis when gravity and external forces are being placed on those structures to prevent rotation. Without those muscles, we may lose our alignment. They help maintain torso position during movement.

Multifidus

The multifidus is a group of muscles that runs from the base of the spine (sacrum) to the neck (cervical spine) (figure 2.5*a*). They are little sections of muscles that provide segmental stability to the spine. They span in chunks of two to four vertebrae and are key in supporting the back during movement. I tend to focus a bit more on the lumbar fibers in my practice. Some studies have found additional fatty deposits surrounding this tissue in instances of low back dysfunction, indicative of weakness or inhibition. Fat infiltration in the lumbar multifidus (regardless of overall body fat percentage) is higher in those with low back pain (Prasetyo et al. 2020). For many of my clients with low back pain, I check this muscle to ensure it's firing, firing well, and working in integrated movement. Large global movements such as squats, lunges, and rows will all strengthen the multifidus; however, spending time to prime and activate this muscle before loading has, in my experience, been effective.

Dr. Kathy Dooley, anatomist, chiropractor, creator of Immaculate Dissection, and professor shares, "The primary significance of multifidus is to stabilize the lumbar lordosis for spinal cushioning when ambulating. This encourages even weight distribution through the lumbar facet joints and intervertebral symphyseal disc joints, allowing protection for discs and spinal nerve levels traveling to the lower extremity." These muscles act as back stabilizers and support when walking.

Psoas

The psoas is a hip flexor and plays a role in moving the leg forward in the gait cycle (figure 2.5*b*). It also assists to turn the thigh outward and to bend your body sideways in lateral trunk flexion. It has attachments on the lumbar spine (the bony parts of the vertebrae and in the space between the vertebrae called the intervertebral discs), which is why it's placed here in the stabilizer category despite it also playing a role in stabilizing the lumbo-pelvic region. Many focus on stretching the psoas, which can be helpful to relieve tight hip flexors. In my experience, I often find through manual muscle testing and movement screens that this muscle needs strengthening. Adding in loaded hip-flexion-based exercises while maintaining a stable pelvis can ensure this muscle is working well overall.

Gluteus Medius

This muscle's main action is hip abduction or moving the leg away from the body in a sideways motion (figure 2.4). It also stabilizes the pelvis in the frontal plane (e.g., jumping jacks) or ensures the hips remain level and supported during movement, especially in ambulation. Without this stability, the hip may drop or sink when walking as the opposite back foot leaves the ground.

You may have heard of various exercises to work this muscle. The clamshell, a side-lying hip-opening exercise, is a very popular one. This can be a good starting point for some. The goal, however, is to challenge this muscle while standing. Working it with your feet on the ground allows you to build that functional crossover from lying to standing and walking. We'll review some upright, ground-based gluteus medius exercises in chapter 9.

Scapular Stabilizers

Several muscles work together to stabilize the shoulders and ensure that our shoulder blades, rib cage, neck, and shoulders all work harmoniously, allowing for movement when needed and stability when needed. These muscles include the trapezius muscles (figure 2.2). The upper trapezius muscles elevate the scapula (or shoulder blade) (shrugging), the middle trapezius muscles retract the scapulae (squeeze them together), and the lower trapezius muscles depress the scapulae (bring them down). Other scapular stabilizers include the serratus anterior (figure 2.2), which protracts the scapulae (moves them away from each other), and the rhomboids (figure 2.2), which are scapular retractors, scapular elevators, and downward rotators of the scapulae.

Together, the stabilizers of the shoulders maintain their position during movement, allow for smooth motion of the shoulder blades and rib cage, maintain good alignment of the neck and spine, and will be more engaged when walking at faster paces with a more accentuated arm swing.

Foot Intrinsics

Twenty-five percent of the bones, muscles, tendons, and ligaments of the body are housed inside your feet! A great many structures in the foot work to hold us upright and serve as our literal foundation (figure 2.6). The deep muscles of the foot act as shock absorbers and support our body weight. They play a role in overall balance, arch support, and transfer of ground reaction forces. They move the foot and toes in different directions. Challenging these muscles is important to help support our body overall. We'll be touching on the foot in more detail in chapter 3.

Although we mention the muscles individually to highlight specific actions, our body doesn't work in a singular sense. Multiple muscles are integrated in actions like walking. The body works as a whole. While you're extending one hip (glutes, hamstrings, and posterior fibers of the adductor magnus) and plantar flexing the ankle (calves), the same-side arm is moving back into humeral extension (posterior deltoid, latissimus dorsi, teres major), the opposite hip flexor (iliacus, psoas) is pulling the leg forward, and all the core and back muscles are working to stabilize the back and lumbo-pelvic region.

Physiology

The body never ceases to amaze me. The number of complex actions and reactions that take place at a cellular level is astonishing. When things stop working optimally is when we typically realize how comfortable, efficient, and powerful everything is. If you've ever broken a bone, pulled a muscle, sprained an ankle, or sustained an injury that sidelined you in

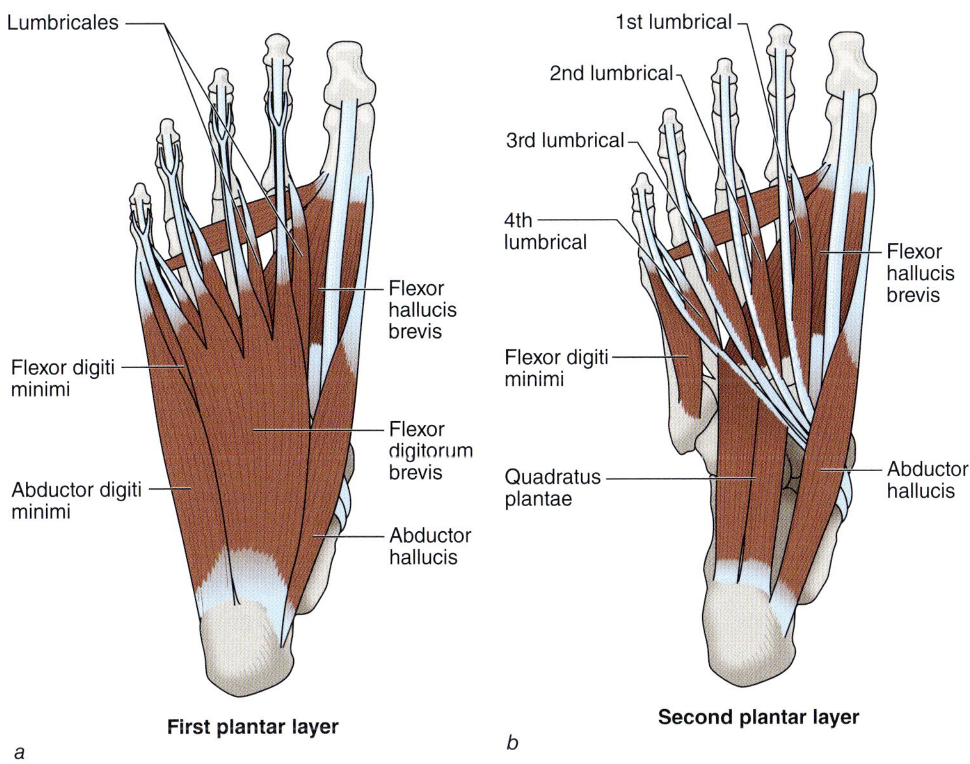

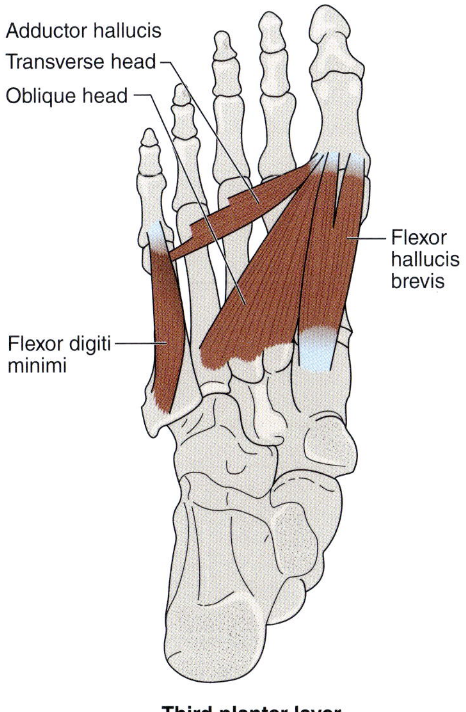

FIGURE 2.6 Deep muscles of the foot: *(a)* first plantar layer, *(b)* second plantar layer, and *(c)* third plantar layer.

any way, you likely identify with the significance of it all. Next, we'll break down just a few of the physiological changes that occur with walking.

Cardiovascular

Walking improves our cardiovascular system efficiently, easily, and conveniently. When moving our limbs, creating contact with the ground, pushing away from the ground with our bodies, and continuing this rhythmic cycle, we are increasing the demand on our heart and other vessels such as arteries, veins, and capillaries. Our respiration rate may increase, our lungs fill up and expel air faster, and our overall output is increased. Our heart rate increases, which leads to improved blood flow and potentially lower blood pressure as a training effect. This challenge trains our cardiovascular system to become more efficient over time. We learned in chapter 1 about the benefits of walking, including reducing the risk of cardiovascular disease.

Skeletal

The load-bearing mechanism of walking builds and maintains bone density. When our foot contacts the ground, our skeletal system works via the muscles, tendons, and ligaments to oppose those forces. The more weight we carry, the harder these structures must work. We build bone via a complex system of breaking down and building up, and the proper nutrients and stimulus are required to ensure we remain in a bone-building state instead of a bone breakdown state. Walking has been proven to maintain and build bone density. A healthy bone state helps prevent bone breaks and fractures and supports the muscles, ligaments, and tendons.

Muscular

We didn't include the muscular system in our first chapter as a potential benefit of walking. However, walking challenges the muscular system, and studies have shown that in older adults, walking helps prevent sarcopenia (muscle loss as we age). Yamada et al. (2015) found that adults over the age of 65 who walked for 6 months increased their muscle mass, especially if they had low muscle mass.

However, for the majority of adults, strength training (in addition to walking and other load-bearing activities) is the gold standard for gaining, maintaining, and strengthening skeletal muscle. Chapter 9 will focus on strength exercise suggestions.

Neural/Motor Control

The body is led by the brain. Walking is a rhythmic activity during which we can focus on different mental tasks other than walking. When walking in obstacle-free environments, we can essentially tune out and let our body take over. This is thanks to the complex neural pathways and signals to and from our brains and muscles that guide us unconsciously. Our spine contains neural networks that respond to signals from our skin, environment, eyes, and more, which will then modify the gait pattern in cooperation with the brain.

The brain needs to adjust and adapt to ensure the body remains in a state of balance while moving. Single-leg stability is important in walking, and including exercises to improve single-leg stability is key to becoming and remaining efficient walkers. We'll often adjust step length and other variables to ensure we're stable and efficient when walking.

Dr. Greg Wells, PhD, physiologist, researcher, professor, and author, emphasizes the importance of movement and mental activation for optimal brain functioning. Sitting for long periods of time impairs our brain's ability to function. We can keep our brain alert and energized by injecting frequent bouts of exercise snacks throughout the day. He shares,

> Think of it as micro-dosing on movement. You will find it makes a huge difference to your attention, creativity, and execution. As little as 15 minutes of exercise improves mental performance, so add this to your day before important tasks that you have to do. If you have an important thinking-related task to do during the day—for example, a presentation, a major meeting, or an exam—try to take a few minutes to do some light exercise before the event. If you need to solve a problem, block off some time to get focused and make sure that you walk, stretch, or lift some weights in the hour before you settle in to work on the challenge. Exercise will increase the flow of oxygen and nutrients to the brain and improve your mental performance. It might seem like you're taking too much time away from the task, but the physiology says that you'll perform better and get healthier at the same time.

Dr. Wells also stresses the importance of mindful movement and moving meditation.

> Moving meditation is any exercise in which you're moving your body in a repetitive pattern, such as walking. Simple movements at a low, consistent intensity allow your mind to relax and de-stress. Leave your headphones elsewhere to be fully present and mindful. The idea is to get into a slow, easy, regular rhythm to the point where you don't have to think much about or assess what you're doing. You want to

experience the flow of your rhythm and pull your thoughts away from "the business of life" to your own experience: how your body feels, how the air smells, and so on. Try to coordinate your breathing with the motion. Be attentive to the movement of your body and your bodily sensations. Let go of your "busy brain."

When we do those types of rhythmic, repetitive activities, we drop into theta brain waves. That's why when we are on a long walk, we start ideating and creating. We come up with new solutions to old problems. You get wellness benefits for mind and body at the same time!

Hormonal

Chen et al. (2022) found that including regular short bouts of brisk walking when sitting for long periods increases postmeal gut hormones. These specific gut hormones may play a role in improving blood sugar management, appetite regulation, and obesity. In older adults, walking can increase anabolic (muscle building) hormone levels (Yamada et al. 2015). Walking can also release hormones such as endorphins, our pain-dampening and feel-good enhancements.

In general, the right dose of physical activity helps to ensure our hormones are optimized. Many other factors affect overall hormone health, such as sleep, nutrition, stress, and certain diseases or conditions. For men and women, walking can boost beneficial hormones, which help to regulate several functions such as digestion, heart health, sleep, metabolism, mood, organ health, growth and development, fertility and reproduction, and more.

As we gain a more concrete understanding of our foundations (literally and figuratively), we can move on to understand the different challenges that gear and terrain can provide. Next, we'll provide gear recommendations and discuss how different terrains can affect how we walk.

CHAPTER 3

Gear and Terrain

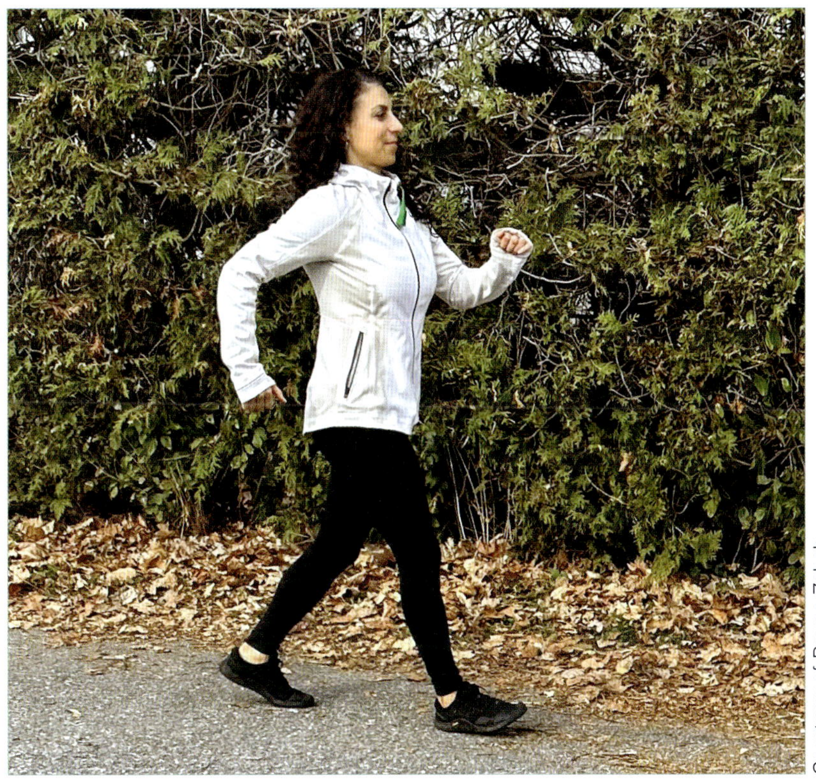

Courtesy of Rayne Zahab.

Gear and clothing can make or break any outdoor activity. If we dress appropriately (with the right fabrics and layers), use tools to help us, and wear the right shoes, we will feel the best on our walks, from head to toes. In this chapter, we'll expand on footwear, clothing, gear, and terrain as well as fuel and hydration to help us put our best foot forward.

Footwear

Walking in proper footwear is essential, and investing in a good pair of walking shoes will provide comfort and support, prevent injury, and more. They should be replaced at regular intervals to ensure they are supporting us as intended. Some experts recommend replacing footwear after a specific amount of time; others recommend replacing shoes after a certain amount of mileage. Roger Burrows, race walking coach, recommends walkers replace their footwear every 400 miles (~650 km). His club members are used to hearing "three pairs of training shoes per year, with at least one extra pair for the more advanced walkers." Ryan Grant, certified pedorthist and owner of Solefit, recommends using 500 to 625 miles (~800-1,000 km) as a guide to start looking for unusual wear on the bottom of the shoes or any new injury spots.

Who Should I Consult?

Several health care professionals can help with footwear recommendations and gait analysis. It can be difficult to know who to see first. Although there are foot specialists (such as podiatrists, pedorthists, and chiropodists), there are other health care professionals such as physiotherapists or chiropractors who also may be able to help. It's likely best to start with word of mouth. "Check in with your local running/walking specialty stores and ask them what their recommendation is. Who do they send their walkers to? That would likely be your best start as it's not necessarily about the type of practitioner but more about finding someone who really specializes with working with walkers and gait," shares Ryan Grant.

Selecting the right pair of shoes can be a difficult endeavor. Endless options are available, which can be beneficial, because our feet are individual and our needs differ based on various factors. According to Grant, "there are minimalist shoes, maximalist shoes, hiking shoes, running shoes, walking shoes, and everything in between that all have their place depending on what's needed. For many of us starting a walking program, we grab an old shoe out of the closet and get started with the thought being that we'll invest in a better shoe if the walking program sticks. Unfortunately, the lack of correct footwear can prevent us from establishing that walking program due to injury or lack of comfort."

Considering our goals, intensity, volume, terrain, frequency, and level of injury may all be factors that play a role in the type of shoe required. Grant recommends, "the focus should likely be on giving you the safest shoe to protect you for how you're currently walking. Traditional running shoes tend to be best here. Many of us have spent years wearing higher heeled shoes (dress shoes and casual) along with sitting at work, so the traditional running shoe tends to be more protective to allow someone to get out on the road or trails quicker and safer. Type of terrain a walker will be primarily frequenting will then determine the specifics (i.e., running shoe versus walking shoe versus trail shoe)."

When we plant our heel and roll through our foot, our toes need to splay outward. Wearing a shoe that allows our toes to spread is important. Restricting our toes may lead to foot, ankle, and lower limb issues. Check to see if your shoes are wide enough to allow for natural toe splaying when walking: Remove your insole from your shoe and place your foot directly on it. Spread your toes outward. If your toes stay on the insole, you likely have enough space. If your toes move off the sides of the insole when spreading them, they are likely not wide enough. Feet are meant to be widest at the end of the toes and not the base of the toes. Purchasing a wide shoe is not always indicative of a good fit. Ideally, you're looking for shoes that fit the shape of your foot.

The foot contains 33 joints, 26 bones, and over 100 muscles, tendons, and ligaments! These muscles need to be loaded and strengthened similar to other muscles. When we constantly wear supportive footwear indoors and outdoors, our feet have a limited ability to be strengthened and challenged. According to Grant, "these shoes can also enable some bad habits due to the fact that they tend to be more protective with their more elevated heel, extra cushioning, and support. That's where a more minimalist shoe might come into play to allow the feet to work a bit more (like taking your feet to the gym). These shoes are often flatter and more flexible to allow your feet to do more of the work. We're humans, and as such we are miraculously designed to be barefoot, which is why this type of footwear can be great."

Curtis et al. (2021) found that daily activity in minimal footwear increases foot strength. Grant warns, "however, most people aren't ready to wear them for very long, so caution is definitely advised with this type of shoe. If someone's goals are to ensure they have their feet working out at the same time as the rest of their body (and want to ensure they're not enabling bad habits), these shoes are great. This, however, comes with a heightened risk of injury and for many will mean they need to initially keep their mileage lower." According to a review by Franklin et al. (2015), those who walked barefoot habitually had lower peak plantar pressures. Lower plantar pressures allow us to reduce pressure on specific areas of our feet. Although other tools may assist in reducing plantar pressure, spending some time walking barefoot indoors, if pain free and tolerable in small doses to start, may be a beneficial strategy to help offload the pressures in our feet and build intrinsic foot strength. Although it has taken me years to work up to, I personally prefer being barefoot or in socks when indoors and alternate between different minimal style shoes when outdoors. Gradually building up to a more minimal shoe will take time and purposeful progression, but it may be of value in the long term with regard to overall foot health.

"When trying to determine the best footwear for you, it's always worthwhile checking in with a professional to give you the peace of mind that you're investing in the correct shoes for you," Grant shares. "Look on local forums to see what shoe stores specialize in working with walkers and runners. Also check to see if there are any pedorthists, podiatrists, physiotherapists, etc., who might specialize in footwear and gait analysis."

Clothing

Clothing needs will change depending on various factors. The temperature, season, humidity levels, intensity, terrain, desired comfort, and time of day will all play a role in deciding what to wear. In general, it's best to wear clothing made of fabric that wicks moisture away from the body. Performance fabrics have changed significantly over the years, and we now have a multitude of options for performance wear. Polyester blends, stretch fabrics, wool blends, and natural and synthetic fabrics are all quite advanced in terms of function, durability, and comfort. Layering in colder temperatures and wearing cooling fabrics in warmer temperatures is ideal.

In colder climates, start with a base layer that retains heat yet moves moisture away from the body. From there, you can layer various pieces depending on the temperature and the intensity of your walk. Slower walks may require warm, dense coats, yet faster paces may require light running jackets. It may take some time to experiment with your best layering strategy. Invest in high-quality fabrics, tested designs, and clothing you feel comfortable in.

In moderate climates, aim for what feels best for you. Your needs may change depending on the time of year, location, temperature, humidity levels, and intensity. If walking on trails or wooded areas with a higher concentration of ticks or other disease-carrying insects, long pants and long sleeves may prevent insect bites. If walking in more shaded areas, early in the morning, or later at night, bring or wear an extra layer. If walking in the middle of the day, during summer months, and on days with a higher UV index, wear cooling and protective fabrics.

In warmer climates, using multiple heat and sun protection strategies is ideal. Hats, sunglasses, clothing with added SPF protection, lighter colors, and a hydration pack may be your best tools. Wearing the correct sun protection and reapplying will help protect you from sun damage. Adjusting walking times, walking intensity, and hydration may be required on hotter days.

Wearables

I distinctly remember a client telling me in 2012 that wearable activity trackers were the future. At the time, they were just becoming popular and were fairly new gadgets. Now, it's hard to imagine a time without them. Using a wearable can have numerous benefits. We can track our steps, heart rate, intensity, sleep patterns and quality, number of calories burned, and more. The objective data can be a strategic motivator for many. If you're someone who's driven by numbers, metrics, and having concrete goals, this may be important and a key driver for you.

Ferguson et al. (2022) suggested that activity trackers improved physical activity and fitness. On average, participants were walking about 40 extra minutes per day while using them. For some, using a wearable device can be motivating; others may not notice a difference at all. Understand your personal drivers. What motivates you? If wearing an activity tracker is key to your success, using one will be beneficial. If exercising in groups, signing up for a race, or creating a reward system motivates you, use that to your advantage. Are you someone who is intrinsically motivated? Follow that intuition. Recognizing that we are all unique and different and using the tools and strategies that help support our individual goals and health can be a strategic advantage.

Lighting, Visibility, and Safety

After a few near misses, I discovered the importance of being seen at night. Even with good street and sidewalk lighting, it can be difficult for vehicles to see pedestrians at dusk and when it's dark out. Use various tools to ensure you're visible and safe, especially at night. Choosing reflective shoes, clothing, and packs can boost visibility. Small lights hooked onto backpacks and sweater or coat zippers can be helpful (figure 3.1). There are also lights that strap onto your arm (figure 3.2). If you're

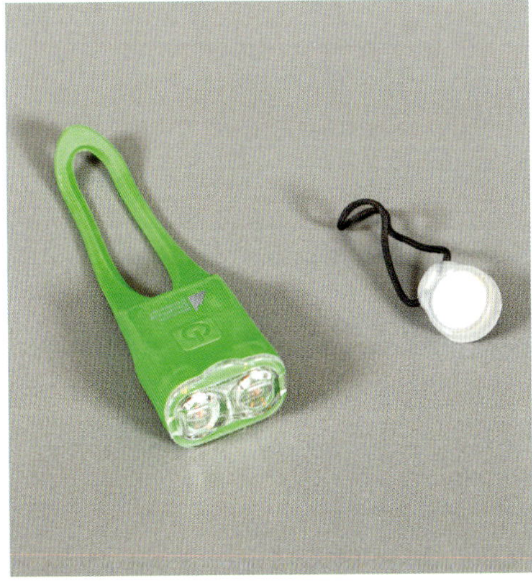

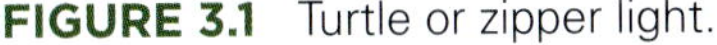

FIGURE 3.1 Turtle or zipper light.

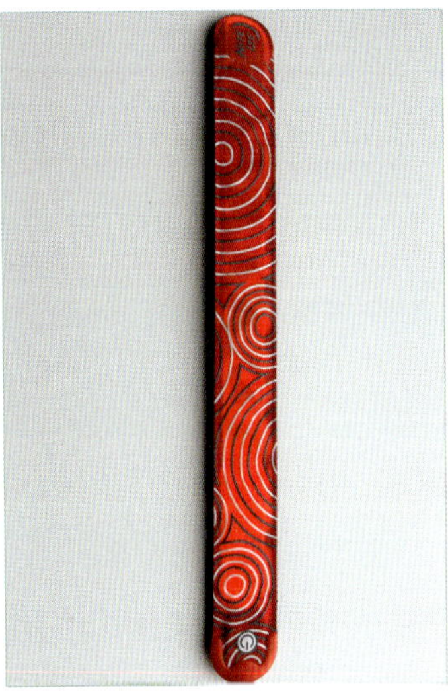

FIGURE 3.2 Wrap light.

walking with a dog at night, use a collar light on your pet so both of you remain visible, no matter the terrain. Most of these tools have options for constant or flashing lights.

Packs

For some of us, wearing a pack to carry items is a necessary tool. Longer walks, hikes, and adventures mean we may need to carry our gear. Items like food, water, extra clothing or socks, supplements, tools, lights, and more may all need to be stored conveniently. There are many options for pack sizes, supports, materials, and reflective safety features. On shorter, faster walks, I will often use a running belt to carry essentials (e.g., phone, ID, keys) and find it more comfortable than placing items in pockets (figure 3.3). On cooler days, pockets in coats, pants, and sweaters may do the trick. On warmer days, the belts tend to provide that ability to walk freely without any restrictions and may be an option for those who want to pack light yet carry essentials while walking briskly.

Posture, support, comfort, function, purpose, size, and convenience are all elements to consider when selecting the right pack. I would recommend consulting with store representatives, trying on various packs, and selecting the one that works best for you from a comfort and practical perspective. Whichever pack you choose, walk with good posture while wearing it. We'll cover posture and alignment in more detail in chapter 4.

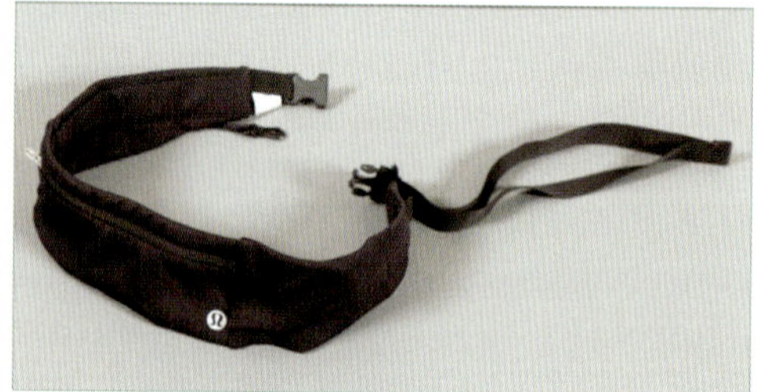

FIGURE 3.3 Running belt.

Terrain

The surface on which we walk will play a role in our comfort, muscle activation, safety, and support. Adding in a variety of different walking surfaces where possible can help to avoid overuse injuries, challenge different muscles, and allow our bodies to adapt to varying environments. Next, we'll discuss several walking surfaces and how they may affect our walks.

Cement or Pavement

For many, most of our walks occur on sidewalks, side streets, and paved pathways. Given the supportive footwear that's available to most of us, these surfaces work well. It's convenient, stable, often clear and safe, easy to maneuver, and suitable for walking with others. Although walking too fast too soon on harder surfaces may lead to injuries and discomforts such as shin splints, walking on pavement and cement is the only option for many. Build volume and intensity slowly, progressively, and purposefully to ensure your muscles, ligaments, and tendons adapt to the increased demand. Staying within your threshold will ensure you continue to walk comfortably for progressively longer periods. It's difficult to go from walking 10 minutes to 100 minutes in a short period of time. Allowing our tissues time to respond will help our bodies build resiliency.

Sand

Something about walking on a sandy beach next to a body of water in ideal weather conditions gives us that perfect hit of endorphins. Although more challenging, it can be rejuvenating and refreshing. Walking on sand requires 1.6 to 2.5 times more mechanical work than walking on hard surfaces at the same speed. Additionally, walking on sand requires 2.1 to 2.7 times more energy expenditure than walking on hard surfaces at the same speed (Lejeune et al. 1998). Overall, walking on the beach or a sandy surface uses more muscle recruitment and energy.

Walking over dry sand will also significantly reduce walking speed (Leicht and Crowther 2007). Although we're working harder, walking slower, and using more muscles and energy overall, many of us still enjoy a leisurely stroll along a beach. It's not uncommon to see people, couples, or children walking and playing along a shoreline. Just the thought of it can bring a sense of calm, remembering how pleasant the sand feels under our feet, how we feel in those environments, and how comfortable our bodies can feel when walking on a sandy surface.

Adding a barefoot element incorporates a whole new dimension of grounding or earthing, where the electrical charges from the sand can have positive effects on the body. It's no wonder we feel refreshed and invigorated after a trip to the beach, whether it's a local beach or midwinter escape to a warm destination.

Forest, Hiking Trails, and Gravel

For some, walking in a forested area can be a spiritual escape, a place where we can breathe deeply, shed our worries, and be at peace with ourselves and those around us. I tend to prefer walking in areas that are more natural. A hiking trail, wooded area, or off-beaten path can be rejuvenating and give us a boost that's hard to replicate. As long as the trails and paths are safe, it offers great variety from an environmental and challenge standpoint. Walking on complex surfaces is associated with a lower head pitch or position, increased muscle coactivation, and reduced walking smoothness (Thomas 2020). Our entire bodies react to different surfaces, and our muscles and head position will change depending on how stable we feel.

Just like walking on a beach, walking on a trail with uneven surfaces will also give us that hit of endorphins. It is a great reset. Many will crave it. It's a difficult emotion to explain, but those who walk on trails and in forests or wooded areas will tell you it's something they just need. It completes their day, offers variety in their environments, and gives them a chance to breathe deeply and connect with nature on a different level. As long as you're in a safe environment, are not getting lost (speaking from personal experience here), and are well equipped for the terrain with proper clothing, footwear, water, and fuel, it can be an uplifting experience.

Hills and Stairs

Walking on an incline provides excellent opportunities for propulsion and powering up. Walking up stairs increases our level of exertion, challenges our muscular and cardiovascular systems, and adds variability and balance to our overall fitness routines. Depending on the number of flights, walking up stairs can bring us to a vigorous level of exercise while remaining low impact. And, depending on the slope and length of a hill, we can observe similar challenges and benefits. Those who walk will often find it challenging to increase their heart rates. Hills and stairs are complementary activities that give everything a boost, remain low impact, yet still challenge all our systems.

Once we anticipate a change in the slope of a surface, our neuromuscular patterns shift significantly from walking on level surfaces (Gottschall and Nichols 2011). We'll need to adapt our gait; our brains will focus on remaining stable in a dynamic environment, and we'll shift the placement of our limbs. Yet, it's a good challenge. It's important to walk on varied surfaces, train our bodies to work in different environments, and load our muscular systems in different ways. This helps us adapt to all situations, creates a resilient system, and ensures we have the capacity for (almost) anything that may come our way.

Get Outside

Although walking indoors on treadmills, indoor tracks, or indoor community spaces has benefits such as safety, accessibility, and stability, walking outdoors has numerous benefits as well. Outdoor exercise can improve mental and physical health as well as boost our overall mood. Outdoor exercise can improve our immune systems, especially in children who play outdoors (Bento and Dias 2017). Those who visit natural spaces weekly are more likely to engage in environmentally friendly behaviors (Deville et al. 2021). We also know that walking outdoors increases creativity (Oppezzo and Schwartz 2014). When it's safe and appropriate to do so, I encourage outdoor walking to help reap the numerous benefits (quantifiable and unquantifiable) it can offer (table 3.1).

TABLE 3.1 Benefits of Indoor Versus Outdoor Walking

Indoor	Outdoor
Accessible	Accessible
Less impact/stress	More muscle recruitment
Increased variability (treadmill)	Increased input from terrain, environment
Stable climate/temperature control	Cool air/breeze/shade at times
Can be safer/more stable	More balance and stability required
Entertainment/distraction	Boost mood
Air quality	Air variable
Focus on form without distractions	Economical
Control over workouts	Increased variety

Treadmill

While I'm a big proponent of walking outdoors, there are certainly benefits to walking indoors, whether on treadmills, indoor tracks, or in community spaces. Walking on a treadmill can provide numerous benefits. It is safer if the conditions outdoors are unsafe due to cold, ice, snow, heat, humidity, air quality, construction, or noise levels. It can also provide greater control over workouts with incline and speed control at your fingertips. For those who travel and prefer to walk indoors, the treadmill in the hotel gym can be a great option if you're unfamiliar with your surroundings. Choosing the treadmill over outdoor walking may provide you with the convenience of fitting a walk in if you have young children and prefer to walk while they nap. For many it can just be easier to listen to a podcast, your favorite music, or tune in to a show while walking inside. I have some high-performing clients who prefer using the treadmill to ensure the speed, time, and incline are exact to allow for consistent and specific training. There are numerous reasons for choosing to walk on a treadmill, and for many, it can be a very worthwhile investment.

Remaining consistent is what's critical for overall success. Doing short, frequent walks can be beneficial. Someone walking or exercising more frequently will typically see greater results than someone walking or exercising inconsistently. If the treadmill provides an option that allows you to remain consistent over time, it's a strategic and key player in your overall results. Do what allows you to remain consistent in the long run. For some, a combination of indoor and outdoor walking will be just that.

From a form and physiological perspective, walking on a treadmill will be different from walking on stable surfaces. During the gait cycle, when we strike our foot on the ground, we have to roll through the foot and push the ground away from us to propel forward. When working on stable surfaces, we use our muscles a great deal to provide that forward action. When we strike our foot on a treadmill, there will be less of a push-away aspect. The treadmill is moving the ground for us; therefore, we use our muscles less to propel us forward. However, in the long run, consistency is what is most important for the majority of us; if the treadmill allows for that regularity, the difference in muscle recruitment would be minimal overall. Where possible, combining indoor and outdoor walks provides greater balance from a physiological perspective.

Hydration and Fuel

A large portion of our bodies is made up of water. We must consume water daily to survive and function optimally. Water is a vital nutrient to cellular health. It is a temperature regulator, a transporter of food metabolites, a waste flusher, a shock absorber, a joint lubricator, and a saliva former. It's essential to life. Dehydration will affect numerous systems including our digestion, organs, skin, and more. We can live for periods of time without food, but we cannot survive long without water.

Our specific hydration demands will vary depending on body size, environmental conditions, physical activity, and sweat rate. Drinking more on days where we sweat more due to increased physical activity or heat is important. Drinking before and after activity is wise, and depending on the length, level of exertion, and temperature, drinking during walks may be valuable.

As someone who stands and moves for a good portion of the day, I personally find I feel best having water throughout the day. Others may prefer to have fluids with snacks and meals. I would recommend finding the hydration strategy that works best for you to ensure you're remaining well hydrated. Please consult with your primary health provider or registered dietitian for more guidance.

Fueling one's body daily with sufficient nutrients is very individual. "Energy balance, eating behaviors and food choices tend to differ by type of physical activity, exercise, or sport one is doing, physical performance goals as well as by health goals," according to sports dietitian Dr. Elizabeth Mansfield. Mansfield recommends fueling for the work that is required. "Focus on eating plant-based protein rich foods more often, include a variety of vegetables with meals, and snack on fruits more often. Choose minimally processed foods such as whole grains, plain milk and yogurt, and plant-based proteins such as natural nut butters, and cooked legumes (chickpeas, black beans, lentils, etc.). Limit mass-produced, ready-to-eat packaged foods with low-cost ingredients such as sugary drinks, cereals and snack bars, chips and other snack foods (frozen meals, luncheon meats, etc.). These hyperpalatable foods increase your energy intake and lead to diets high in fats, sugars, and salt (sodium) but low in key nutrients one needs for optimal health and performance."

Protein, carbohydrates, and unsaturated fats are essential. Eating a variety of high-quality food sources of these nutrients will help improve our overall well-being and ensure we get the essential vitamins and minerals required for optimal health. Including protein-rich foods, whether animal or plant based, at every meal and after a walk or workout is key for muscle remodeling and repair. Carbohydrate-rich foods such as grains and cereals, and sources of healthy unsaturated fats found in foods such as nuts, seeds, and avocado provide us with energy for all our daily physical activities, exercise, and sports.

We also want to be mindful of when we eat. Consuming adequate foods prior to being active will help you feel energetic and walk with vigor. As Boston-area sports dietitian Nancy Clark states, "Walkers who make breakfast and lunch their main meals of the day will likely enjoy higher energy walks than those who skimp on those meals. Walkers want to fuel well during the active part of their day." Clark also shares, "If you find yourself thinking a lot about food during your walks, you likely are hungry. Hunger is a simple request for fuel. Getting too hungry triggers cravings for sugar and sweets. To curb cravings for sweets, enjoy satisfying breakfasts and lunches. Walkers who eat enough at those meals will not only boost their energy levels but also curb hunger."

For some, our needs may shift depending on the day, activity level, time of month for women, phase in our life we're in, or specific health goals. "Over time, daily dietary patterns, if deficient in essential nutrients, have a detrimental impact on the overall functioning and health of the human body," according to Mansfield. Often, it takes time to explore and note what is working from a digestive, energy, sleep, mood, and vitality perspective before we narrow down what is ideal for our own bodies. If you're in doubt, please consult with your primary health care provider or registered dietitian to help guide you on your individual nutrition journey.

Now that you're armed with the right gear and fuel and are ready for varying walking surfaces, we'll be breaking down proper breathing and alignment in the next chapter. Our next section on mastering the form of walking will help provide a foundation and base for good walking technique.

PART II

MASTER THE FORM

CHAPTER 4

Breathing and Alignment

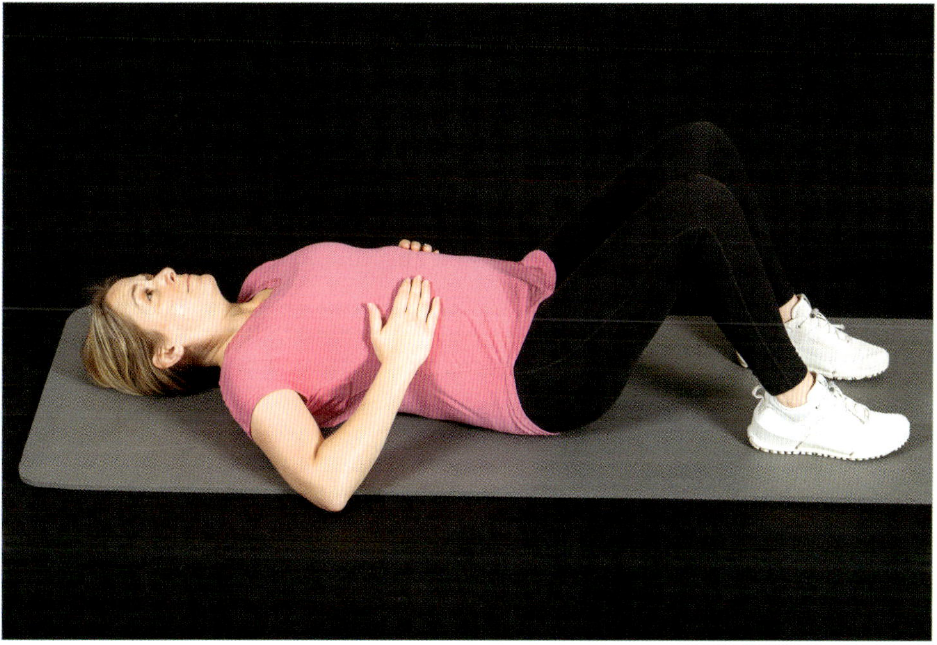

It's common to focus on specific elements such as foot placement, cadence, stride length, and speed when walking. However, alignment and breathing also play a pivotal role in muscle recruitment, walking mechanics, and overall comfort and efficiency when walking. Our alignment and breathing serve as a good base or foundational aspect for us before moving into adding speed or drills. Perfecting our stacked positioning and breathing optimally will bring a bit more comfort and ease to our walks.

Alignment

Breathing and posture are intricately linked. To breathe well, we need good body alignment. Breathing is easier when the body is well aligned. Proper posture and alignment help prevent injury and increase comfort, power, intensity, and longevity. Perfect posture all day isn't required. We ideally want to avoid remaining static in any one posture. Moving into many postures and positions throughout the day helps us to remain mobile, comfortable, and less stagnant. Our best posture is really our next posture. Spending more time in better alignment has a positive impact on the body. It allows us to be more efficient, comfortable, and stable.

No consistent link between body posture and pain exists, but Kim et al. (2015) found that an exercise program for posture correction (performed for 20 minutes, three times per week, for 8 weeks) decreased pain levels, notably in the shoulders, midback, and low back. Not everyone who corrects their posture will feel less pain, but it is worth exploring for some. I often compare alignment to Jenga blocks. When one block moves out from the stack, the stack becomes less stable. As more and more Jenga blocks move out of the stacked position, the support is less and less stable, and at some point, something has to give. Creating a more stacked position when walking places less strain on surrounding muscles and joints. It allows us to use our core muscles more optimally, feel more comfortable, and generate more power and amplitude.

Although spending more time in better posture is helpful, long periods of time stuck in any posture isn't ideal. Allowing for movement when sitting and standing throughout the day is best. I recommend taking frequent movement breaks or snacks and breaking long periods of sitting or standing with some form of dynamic movement (e.g., walking or stretching). If you, like me, spend long periods of time standing or sitting at work, sometimes in awkward postures, posture-specific exercises and stretches will help you feel your best. In my experience, I have fewer headaches, feel less discomfort in my body, and move with more ease and comfort when I include posture-specific exercises and stretches into my weekly routine.

Optimal alignment has the following characteristics (figure 4.1):

1. Head, shoulders, hips, and feet aligned
2. Ear, side of shoulder (acromion process), hip (top of iliac crest), lateral knee, and lateral ankle (lateral malleolus) aligned
3. Ribs stacked over hips (very little to no rib flare)
4. Hips over ankles (iliac crest over lateral malleolus)
5. Weight in midfoot

Postural Imbalances

Many variations of normal posture will allow us to move and perform at our best. Sometimes we move beyond these normal limits and encounter postural imbalances that may affect how we move and feel. A few of these postural imbalances that may affect your comfort and mechanics are

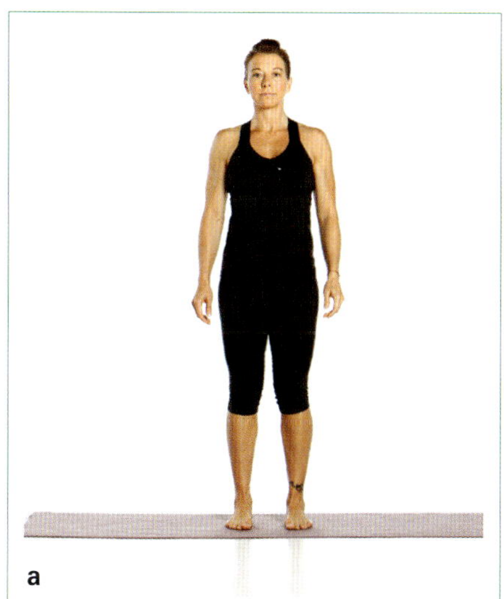
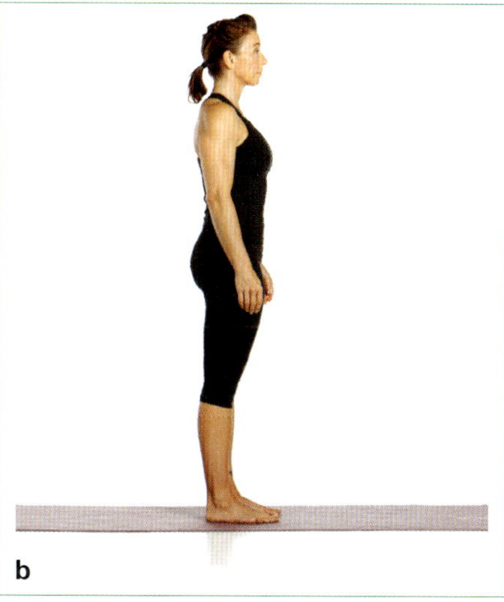

FIGURE 4.1 Optimal alignment: *(a)* anterior view and *(b)* side view.

described next. If you're unsure about your posture, especially if you're experiencing pain or discomfort, reach out to a practitioner who can help assess and correct your positioning, especially during movement.

Rib Flare

Rib positioning is tricky to address. For some, our ribs may be in a rib-flared position (figure 4.2)—that is, ribs not stacked directly over the hips. This rib flare may make it challenging to connect with deeper core muscles. We ideally want our ribs to settle so they stack over our hips without being shifted in a tilted-up position.

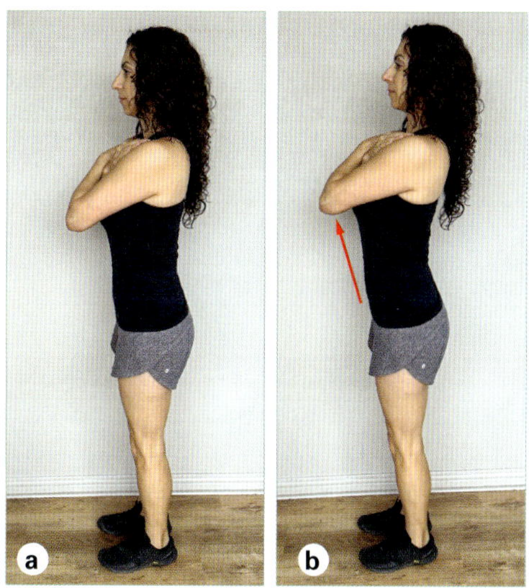

FIGURE 4.2 Rib positioning: *(a)* ideal posture and *(b)* rib flare.
Courtesy of John Zahab.

To see if your ribs flare, try this: Place your fingers on the insides of your hip bones and apply some pressure. You can perform this test in a seated or lying down position. Exhale forcefully to feel your deep core muscles engaging. Now, try it again with your ribs flared out and up. Notice a difference? Stack your ribs over your hips and exhale again. You'll feel more of a core activation with the proper rib or hip alignment. When the diaphragm is positioned directly over the pelvic floor, the transversus abdominis and deeper core muscles can fire optimally. If we're walking with our ribs tilted upward, our core may not work as well to support us, no matter how hard we contract those muscles.

Overcorrecting

Sometimes we try hard to correct our posture and end up overcorrecting (figure 4.3). This may lead to overextending our backs and putting us out of alignment in the opposite direction. A wall can help us feel our body positioning and prevent overcorrection. Stand back against a wall with your feet slightly away from the wall and your knees slightly bent. Place your hips, low ribs, shoulders, and head against the wall. Ensure your chin is parallel to the floor. If your head doesn't touch the wall with your chin level with the floor, move your head back gently while keeping your chin parallel. The chin should not jut up to the ceiling because that is extending the neck. Feel the well-aligned body position and step away from the wall, aiming to keep this alignment for a while. Try walking around a bit with this checked posture and see how it compares to your standard posture. What needs to change or shift?

Pick one element to work on at a time. If the head, shoulders, and ribs are out of alignment, pick one to focus on and work on that element for a week or so until it feels comfortable. Once that element feels more natural, add in another challenge and work on that until you feel comfortable. For some, starting with the head position has a positive trickle-down effect, and for most, it is a beneficial starting point. Come back to the wall every so often to check in and reset. The wall keeps us from overcorrecting our posture and reminds us of better positioning.

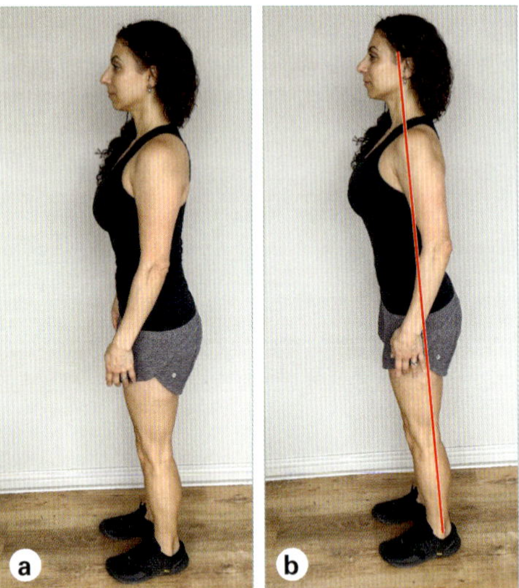

FIGURE 4.3 Posture: *(a)* ideal and *(b)* overcorrected.
Courtesy of John Zahab.

Posture Setup

1. Stand with your back against a wall with your feet a few inches away from the wall and your knees bent.
2. Place your hips, ribs, shoulders, and head against the wall (chin parallel).
3. Step away from the wall, aiming to keep your well-aligned position.
4. Use the wall periodically to reset posture throughout the day if needed (figure 4.4).

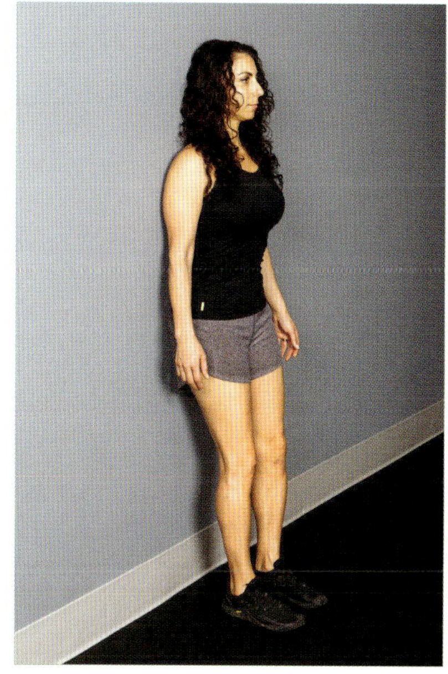

FIGURE 4.4 Posture setup on wall.

Hinging Back at Thoracolumbar Junction

One common postural correction I make includes lengthening the back line to become a bit smoother. I will often see people hinging back at their thoracolumbar (T/L) junction, where the thoracic spine meets the lumbar spine, around the waistline (figure 4.5*a*). This joint is where many extend backward (think of someone holding a baby and leaning back or reaching an arm back to throw a ball), and the setup often pulls us into a leaning back posture (or hinging back at the T/L junction). This posture may give the appearance of looking like someone is in an anterior pelvic tilt—that is, when the pelvis tilts forward, creating a more pronounced low back curvature. Some individuals may be told that they are in an anterior pelvic tilt because their back has the appearance of being in an excessive lumbar curvature. For some, however, the correction needs to occur higher up the back and not necessarily at the hips/pelvis. If we're leaning back (imagine holding a baby), we want to focus on coming forward, stacking our ribs over our hips and straightening our backs versus tucking the pelvis under. Tucking the pelvis under, especially if we are not in an anterior pelvic tilt or sway back posture, may take the pelvis out of neutral and add to (potentially more) glute gripping (see chapter 9). This hinging back posture may place additional strain on the lumbar spine and muscles, and smoothing out that back line by pulling the ribs down, lengthening the back, and imagining the head being pulled straight up to the ceiling may help realign, shift pressures, and potentially take some load off the back (figure 4.5*b*).

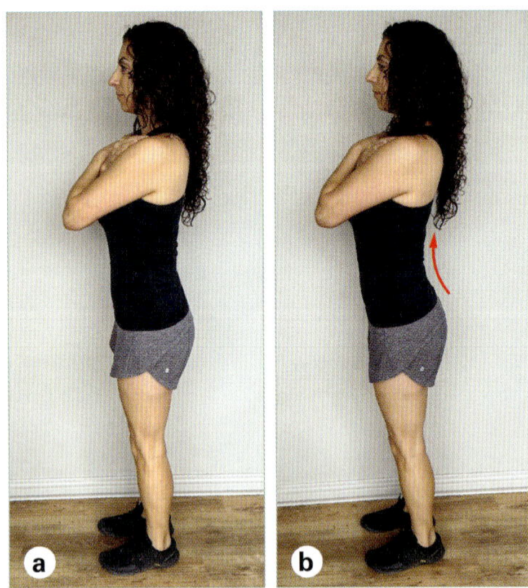

FIGURE 4.5 Hinging back at T/L junction posture: *(a)* ideal posture and *(b)* hinged posture.
Courtesy of John Zahab.

To correct this hinged position, stand with your back against the wall and pay special attention to the low ribs. Are they touching the wall? If they are off the wall, gently press them back against the wall to smooth out the back line. This correction may also help with a rib flare.

We can also try the correction in a supine position on the floor. Lie on your back with your knees bent. Place your hand under your low ribs. Is there a lot of space? Bring the low ribs to touch the ground without tucking your pelvis. You're aiming to dissociate the pelvis and the thoracic spine separately. A gentle exhale or small cough may help. You can also think of performing an abdominal crunch without lifting your head, to bring the ribs closer to the ground.

Alignment With Walking

As we move through our walking pattern, we want to maintain as much of this optimal positioning as possible. Walking is a dynamic form of movement, and our postures will shift and change with each step. Jaime Sochasky Livingston, Certified Athletic Therapist and cofounder of Neuro Reconditioning and the educational company ReconditioningHQ.com, shares this:

> A good walking posture presents as proper alignment through the foot/ankle, knee, hip on one side with the pelvis and torso/spine, and the opposite side upper limb swing providing an efficient body position in space and effective control and coordination of the center of gravity. On a single leg, the pelvis and spine can be said to be

maintained as an inverted "T" (figure 4.6) when in an efficient walking posture. This allows for efficient limb dissociative movement, having a stacked trunk/cylinder positioning to provide anchors for our limbs, and helps to optimize good breathing and efficient joint motion.

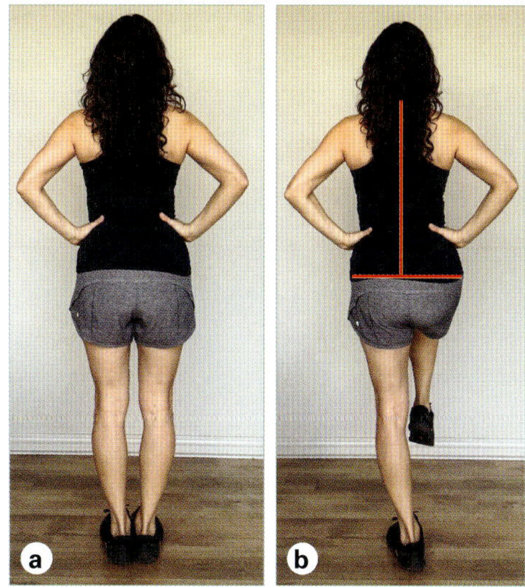

FIGURE 4.6 Inverted T.
Courtesy of John Zahab.

The brain is a key component to consider when it comes to walking. Movement is governed by the brain, and walking posture is reflexive in nature. Sochasky Livingston explains:

> Walking is a pattern that resides in the procedural memory area of our brain. That is to say that 99.9 percent of our standing and walking posture is controlled reflexively. To have efficient and effective standing and walking motion, our reflexes, and the centers that provide feedback to the brain, must be optimal as well. The areas to be maintained and optimized are those that control our brain's sense of itself in space, its ability to coordinate the body relative to gravity, and the visual field and interpretation of the surrounding environment.
>
> For example, as a person ages, they often begin to bend forward, which can be due less to a weakness or postural habit and due more to a lack of peripheral vision, as bending forward allows the visual field to cover the ground better in front of their feet. Hence, by improving their peripheral vision, their body will often no longer need to reflexively bend forward, their posture will improve and, by extension, so will their walking efficiency. By improving any of the feedback areas and reflexes you can help improve the overall pattern. An efficient walking motion will look smooth, with an upright torso, and has rhythmic, balanced, dynamic limb motion and smooth breath pattern.

Our brain and bodies need coordinated efforts to produce smooth, efficient motion. Most of the time, the signals and pathways are clear and connected. If we're experiencing pain, discomfort, difficulties with balance, or changed walking patterns and symmetry, seeking professionals to assess and provide care, including visual and vestibular drills, may be helpful. Pay attention to alignment during strength exercises, which supports and reinforces optimal positioning. In chapter 9, we'll explore various strength exercises to help support and strengthen our bodies. Setting up our alignment and posture well before we start will be key.

Breathing

We inhale and exhale roughly 22,000 times per day. We assume that because we're breathing, we're breathing right, right? Sometimes our breathing mechanics can alter intra-abdominal pressures and lead to imbalances, tightness, pain, and discomforts in the body. Starting with proper breathing helps cardiovascular exercises feel more efficient and easeful, may improve alignment, and can have many mental and physiological benefits. This section will describe proper breathing mechanics, common breathing dysfunctions, and tips and strategies to improve overall breathing.

Breathing Mechanics

The foundation for proper breathing begins with good alignment. When we're well aligned, breathing becomes more efficient and easeful. A well-stacked system allows for good pressure distribution and filling. In proper breathing mechanics, we want to think of filling up our lungs with air on each inhale, similar to filling up a balloon. To take a full, deep breath, we need our rib cage to expand to give our lungs the extra space it requires for the uptake of oxygen. Our internal pressure or intra-abdominal pressure is effectively managed with our diaphragm, muscles, body positions, and breathing mechanics as well as other factors. When our ribs don't expand laterally (or in a 360-degree fashion), it's like squeezing a balloon on the sides. Our intra-abdominal pressure gets shifted up, down, front, or back, placing additional pressures on other areas such as the back, abdominal wall, or pelvic floor. Filling just the chest or just the belly does not allow us to take a full, deep breath, despite the many touted benefits of belly breathing. The lungs are housed in the rib cage, not in the belly or upper chest. We're aiming to breathe more diaphragmatically, allowing all the ribs to move and the diaphragm to open and piston downward, helping to modulate and manage intra-abdominal pressures more efficiently. We want the belly and ribs to move and shift, as well as the chest, in small amounts in a balanced fashion.

Break that down by trying this:

1. Lie on your back with your knees bent, your spine straight, your chin parallel to the wall, and your ribs level with your hips. Watch that your ribs are not jutting upward; try to feel all your ribs along your back making contact with the floor.

2. Place your hands on the sides of your rib cage, with your palms touching your ribs. Your pinky finger is on the lower rib area and your thumb is on the mid- to upper rib area.
3. Take a deep inhale, expand all your ribs outward and backward as well as upward. Think of a balloon filling up with air (in your rib cage, not your belly). Keep your shoulders calm and your neck muscles relaxed. Ideally, we want movement in your belly, ribs, and chest. Some belly and chest movement is okay in inhalation; we want to allow the ribs to make space for the lungs filling up with air.
4. Pause at the top of the inhale for a moment and check to see if you can create more space in the thoracic region (front, side, and back).
5. Exhale slowly, allowing the air to move outward and let your body soften passively as you do so.
6. Repeat for a few minutes daily, allowing this practice to become more comfortable and natural over time.

We want to ensure our breathing strategy matches the demand of our activities. A sprinter needs to have a more robust and strong breathing strategy than someone walking slowly down the street. A breathing strategy too strong may place additional strain on the system and increase the demand of our muscles and respiratory system unnecessarily. A forced, strong breath may help prepare us to lift very heavy objects or run fast but may be unnecessary for day-to-day, easier tasks. We want to soften strategies where possible to create more ease and comfort in our bodies.

This diaphragmatic form of breathing is ideal and more efficient than belly-only or chest-only breathing. Jill Miller, author of *Body by Breath* and *The Roll Model*, shares: "The diaphragm is central to multiple physical and physiological systems of your body. Not only is it the prime mover in respiration, but it also plays a role in posture, digestion, blood and lymphatic flow, sneezing, childbirth, and so much more. Much of its behavior is automatic; you don't need to think about the diaphragm's role in maintaining your life, but when you focus on it and deliberately control its movements, the diaphragm becomes even more functional in its automatic duties." It's important to check in and practice this form of breathing to help support the multiple systems that our breath affects.

Breathing Drills

Before beginning breathing drills, remove any potential obstructions. Tight clothing, straps, or sports bras may impede movement. Clear the sinuses and look for a quiet and comfortable setup. Incorporate breathing drills, tools, and strategies throughout your day.

SUPINE BREATHING

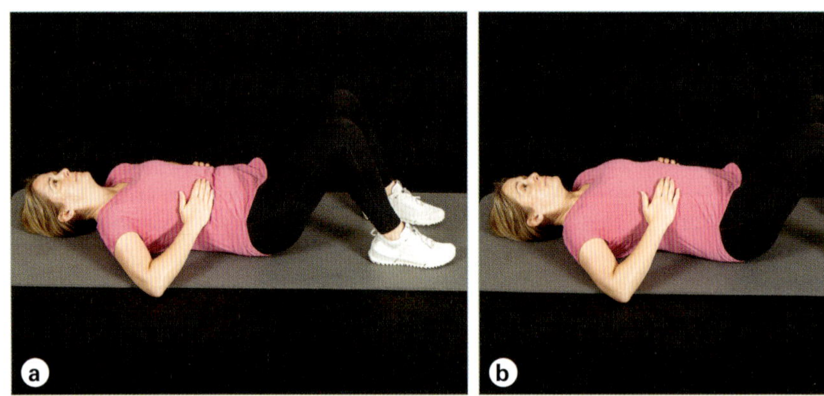

Instructions

Lie on your back with your chin parallel to the wall, your low ribs in contact with the floor, and your knees bent *(a)*. Keep the spine neutral, even if there's a slight curve in the lumbar spine. It's not necessary to push the low back into the floor. Place your hands on your rib cage and inhale deeply, feeling the ribs expand outward into your hands *(b)*. Fill the belly, ribs, and chest at the end of the inhalation while keeping your shoulders and neck relaxed. Exhale fully, allowing the belly to soften and relax.

Variation

Place a band around your rib cage and cross the band in front, holding on to the ends in your hands. Inhale and expand the ribs *(c)*. The band will stretch as you inhale and move the ribs outward. Exhale and return to your start position.

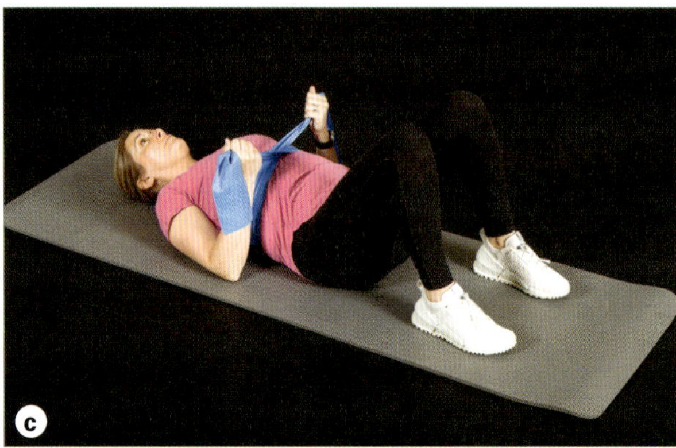

SIDE-LYING BREATHING OVER ROLLED-UP HAND TOWEL

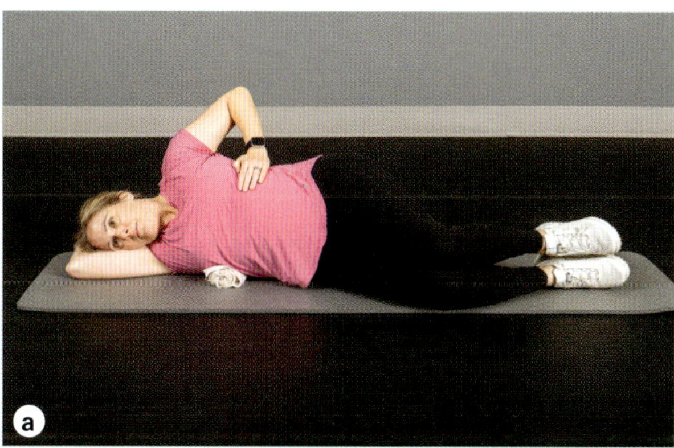

Instructions

Lie on your side with your knees bent and your head, hips, and ankles in line. Your head can rest on a small pillow, a block, or your folded up arm. Place a small, rolled-up towel (hand towel size is appropriate) under your ribs. When the towel is rolled up, it should be about an inch or two in height (maximum). Place your top hand on your rib cage. Inhale deeply and feel the top ribs expanding toward the ceiling; exhale and feel the bottom ribs melting into the rolled-up towel *(a)*. Take a few breaths and move the towel higher on the rib cage. Repeat the breathing a few more times and move the towel up again, stopping just below shoulder level. Repeat on the other side.

Variation

For a deeper stretch, once you've felt the ribs moving outward, move your top arm overhead to stretch out and lengthen your side. Allow the arm to drape over the head as you breathe deeply *(b)*.

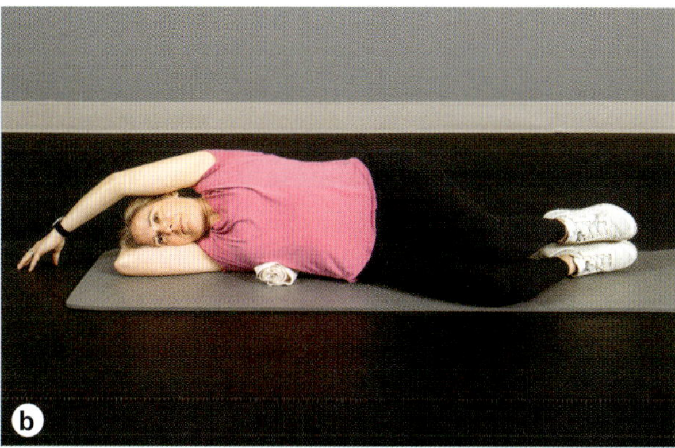

SEATED BREATHING WITH BAND

Just as we become proficient with certain exercises, breathing drills can be progressed as well. We can progress our exercises off the floor to seated and standing postures that closely mimic our day-to-day activities.

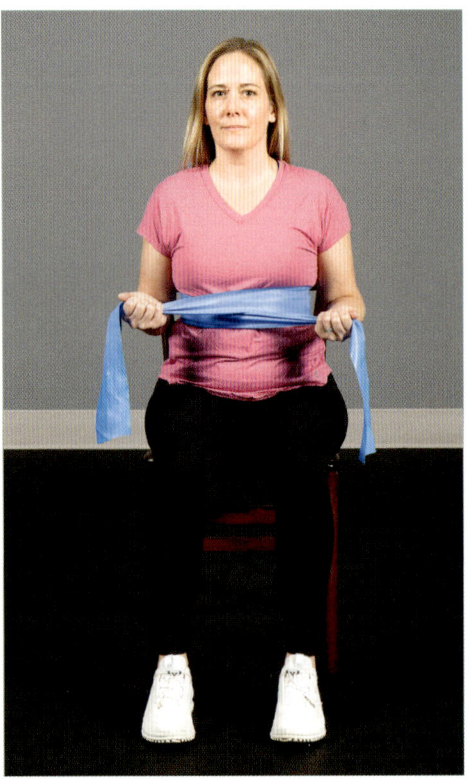

Instructions

Sit or stand tall. Place a TheraBand around the rib cage, with the band crossed in front and our hands holding on to the ends. Inhale and expand into your rib cage, feeling the band move outward as you inhale. Exhale and allow the band to passively return to your start position.

Variation

For a greater challenge, tighten the band around your ribs or use a band with heavier resistance.

DIAPHRAGM VACUUM: THE ULTIMATE DIAPHRAGM STRETCH

This is one of Jill Miller's favorite breathing drills, which she describes as follows.

> The diaphragm is devoid of the normal stretch receptors that we feel in most of our skeletal muscles. When you stretch your quads, you can feel your quads stretching. But when you stretch your diaphragm, you cannot proprioceptively sense the stretching of the diaphragm; rather, you'll notice the tissues surrounding the diaphragm being moved. This feedback from the diaphragm's neighborhood is very helpful as it can inform you about breath-related restrictions that could be limiting your ability to move your ribs, spine, and even notice unconscious muscle bracing throughout your abdomen and back. This strange exercise isolates the stretch of the diaphragm after you've exhaled all of the air in your body. Once that end of the exhale is complete, try stretching your ribs apart as if you're imitating Popeye's barrel chest. If you're doing this action correctly, it will feel like a profound vacuum has gutted your belly; you may even feel a strong suction in your throat as well.

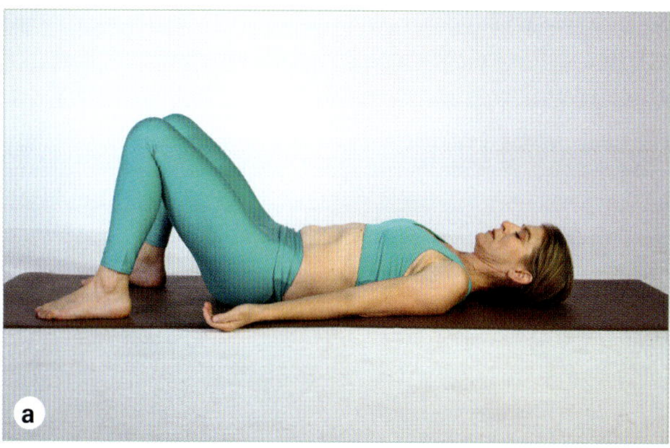

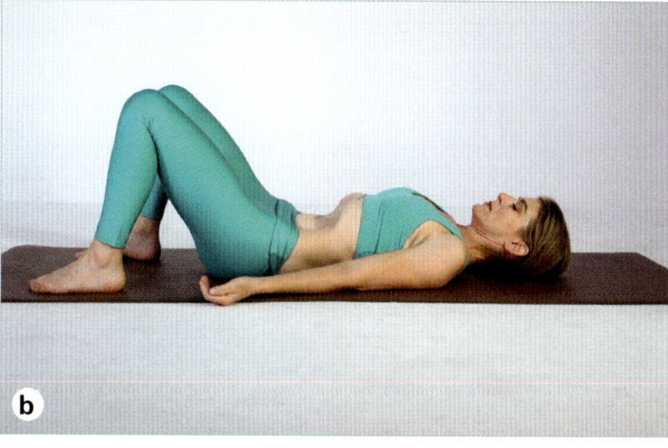

Courtesy of Victory Belt Publishing Inc.

Instructions

Relax on your back and take an abdominal-thoracic breath (complete breath). Exhale completely using the muscles of expiration to empty your lungs. At the end of the exhale, completely relax your abdomen and rib cage *(a)*. Without allowing any air to enter your nose, take a fake inhalation that expands your ribs maximally, creating the shape of a barrel chest. Allow the soft tissues below the rib cage to stretch upward within your body toward the diaphragm and the swelling rib cage *(b)*. Hold the position while you stay calm in the space after exhaling, before you inhale. When your body craves its next breath, release your tensioned rib cage, soften your throat, and then inhale an abdominal-thoracic breath. Repeat for 5 to 8 minutes or for 7 to 20 rounds.

Excerpted by permission from J. Miller, *Body by Breath* (Victory Belt Publishing Inc., 2023).

Breathing Dysfunction (or Suboptimal Breathing Patterns)

A belly-only breathing approach may place additional pressures on the back, abdominal wall, or the pelvic floor. For those with abdominal hernias, diastasis recti, pelvic organ prolapse, or pelvic floor dysfunction (or issues), working to distribute the pressures generated from breathing outward and upward into the ribs and diaphragm may offload the additional strain on the back, abdominal wall, and pelvic floor. A deep belly breath is often touted as beneficial; however, adding in rib expansion and slight chest movement will help this breathing style become complete and efficient.

A chest-only breathing pattern makes it difficult to take deep, full breaths. Our accessory respiratory muscles (the scalenes in the neck and pectoralis minor in the chest) become more active here, leading to an overactivation of the neck and chest muscles. Shifting the breath lower into the ribs and belly can balance out this breathing pattern and allow us to take deeper, fuller breaths.

A paradoxical breathing pattern occurs when the belly pulls inward on inhalation and outward on exhalation. This is opposite to the ideal breathing pattern of expanding and opening when we inhale and a return to neutral when we exhale. Working to relax the neck, core, and pelvic floor without gripping the core may help restore proper breathing mechanics (see "Core Gripping and Glute Gripping" in chapter 9).

Breathing With Movement

Many of us head out the door for our walks, plug in earbuds or find a walking buddy, and go. Breathing is very often the last thing we think of. Most of the time, it's unnecessary to bring extra attention to our breathing patterns while moving. However, a check in every so often can be valuable. Ideally, we should breathe through our noses as much as possible, either in and out or in through the nose and out through the mouth. When the intensity of exercise increases to a certain level, we'll naturally shift to mouth breathing. Practicing more nose breathing throughout the day can filter the air we breathe, boost oxygen uptake, and humidify the air we're taking in. Are we always mouth breathing? Can we breathe through the nose a bit longer, especially with warm-ups and cool-downs? When we shift to mouth breathing, aim to take diaphragmatic breaths as described earlier. Paying a bit more attention to our specific breathing patterns and exploring ways to breathe deeply, more efficiently, and through our noses may help walking feel more comfortable.

Benefits of Breathing Practice

Breathing, meditation, mindfulness, and intentional practices have become more common, even part of our elementary education in many countries. There are countless benefits to breathing, breathing mindfully, and breathing fully and with intention: stress reduction, vagus nerve activation, a sense of peace and calm, quiet minds, to name a few. Zaccaro et al. (2018) found that slow breathing techniques increased feelings of relaxation and alertness and lowered symptoms of anxiety, depression, and anger. Fincham et al. (2023) found that breathwork may be effective for improving stress and mental health.

Sylvie Gouin, author of *Bite-Sized Yoga for Daily Inspiration*, shares this:

> It takes patience, curiosity, and practice to improve our breath, but when we realize that the quality of our breath affects our energy, sleep, and digestion, we are willing to explore. As our greatest source of energy, the breath connects the mind and body. A shallow and fragmented breath and a tense body and stressed mind go hand in hand and, in the same manner, deep and smooth breaths are interconnected with physical and mental ease and vitality. A simple and effective breath visualization is to imagine a bird taking flight when inhaling. Just as their wings expand, our thoracic cavity expands, bringing with it the feeling of vital energy. On the exhalation, as the diaphragm relaxes and returns to its natural dome-shape position, we imagine this bird taking a perch, bringing with it the feeling of calm and stability. Continuing with this visualization for a few

breaths, using inhalation as the source of energy and the exhalation as the source of calm, helps improve the quality of the breath and develops the meditative mind. With practice, we experience that being energized and being calm are intertwined.

Breathing mindfully, diaphragmatically, and through our noses for as long as possible can help us breathe with more ease, efficiency, and comfort. A little bit of practice and awareness goes a long way. In the next chapter we'll discuss gait mechanics and break down the how-to of the walking pattern.

CHAPTER 5

Gait and Walking Technique

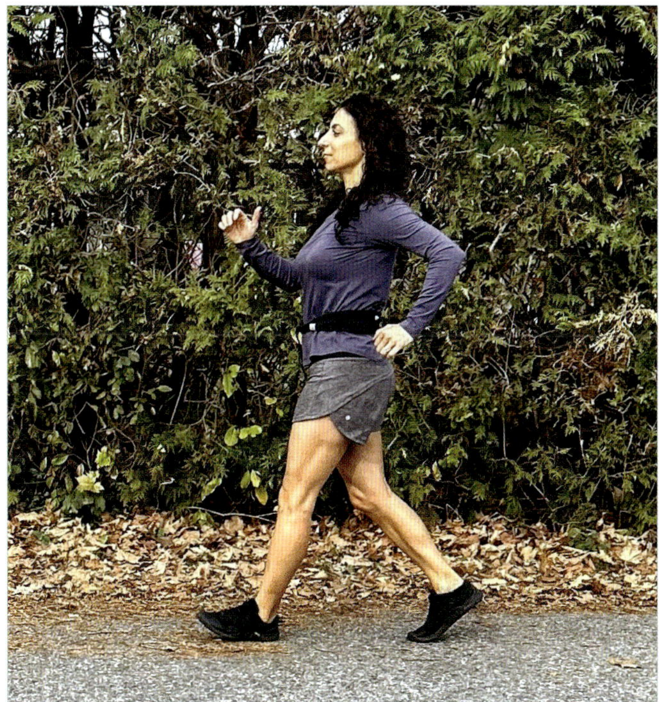

Courtesy of Rayne Zahab.

Our walking gait is like our fingerprints. Many variations of gait fall within normal ranges, yet each person's stepping pattern is unique. Sometimes we can identify someone from afar just by the way they walk. There is no perfect way to walk—we walk in different ways, and it's only a problem if there's a problem. Is there a right way to walk? Yes, and it can look a million different ways. There are more right ways to walk than wrong. Variations are endless and can all be right. It's all about context. If there is dysfunction, we look to correct a pattern to alleviate a symptom or root cause. The only wrong ways to walk are with pain or discomfort. Not every gait is perfect, and we shouldn't strive to be perfect. We should strive to be ourselves and work within in our bodies' parameters. Can we walk more efficiently, however? Absolutely.

If we understand what's within normal ranges, then we know when we should potentially seek out modifications or adjustments to walking form. Understanding our primary objectives when walking can help us as well. Are we going for a leisurely walk with a friend? Am I aiming for a more vigorous workout today? Am I recovering from an injury and using walking as a recovery tool? Is my objective to improve my bone density? We have unique goals when it comes to walking, and our form and intensity may change day to day. Some days we are more energized and can push a little harder, and on other days we may be dragging our feet. That is also normal. Our energy, walking pattern, intensity, volume, duration, and goals will change. It has likely been this way since humans began walking thousands (millions?) of years ago. Keep this in mind as we sift through the information in this chapter.

Phases of Gait

Gait mechanics can be broken into phases. Each phase represents a moment in time when we're landing, absorbing ground forces, and working to propel ourselves forward, to repeat over and over again. Our brain is working proprioceptively to sort out our limb position and muscle actions, all while moving in an automatic sense. In each phase, we can imagine a snapshot of what we ideally want to see and feel. These snapshots together make up our ideal walking blueprint. Figure 5.1 maps out the phases.

Stance phase: Single-leg stability plays a role in this specific phase of walking. Spending time working, balancing, and performing more challenging exercises on one leg will have a functional crossover to walking. About 60 percent of walking is spent in the stance phase. We're ideally looking to move through this stance phase quickly. Once we hit the ground, we don't want to spend too long with our foot sinking into the ground. This allows us to avoid delayed impact forces and decrease our risk of injury. We want to contact, absorb, generate tension, and get off the ground. This allows us to walk efficiently and economically.

1. *Initial contact (heel strike):* We contact the heel first with walking. This phase is when our right foot contacts the ground. Our hips are flexed, our knees are slightly flexed, and our ankles are neutral. The part of the heel striking the ground is ideally the outside of the heel. We often look at our shoes and notice the wear on the outer portion of the heel and believe there is something wrong with our gait pattern when this is actually a normal wear pattern. We want to contact the ground in a slightly more supinated position; this provides more stability

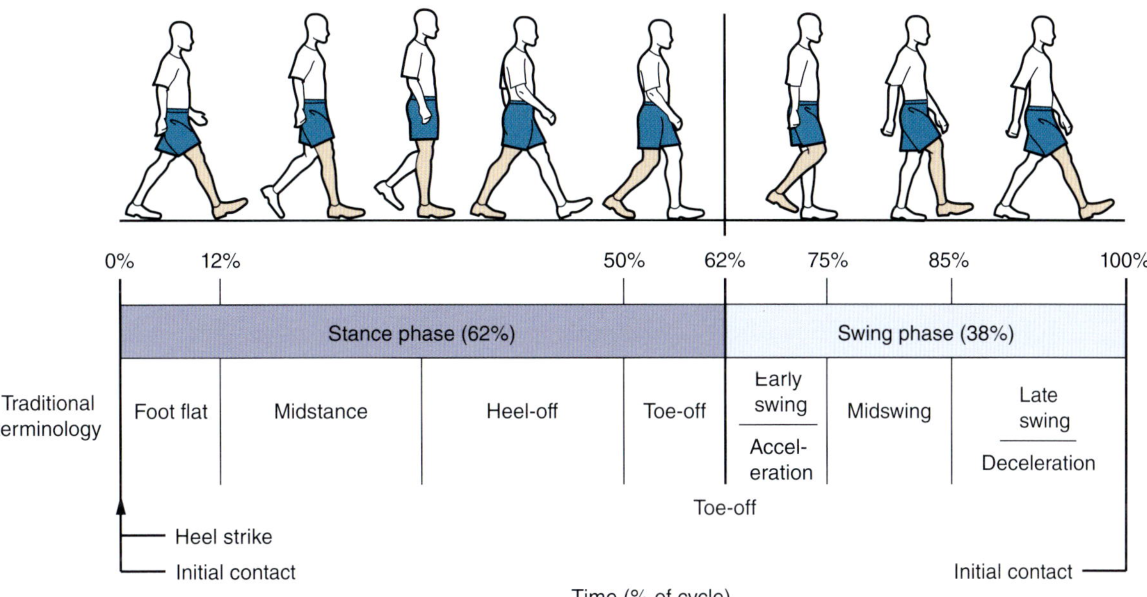

FIGURE 5.1 Phases of gait.

overall, assuming we are absorbing, dampening, and using impact forces to our advantage with our bodies.

We absorb the impact in an isometric manner. Our deep foot muscles contract isometrically to provide stability, stiffness, and splinting in the foot and lower leg. The foot is designed to be stiff when stiffness is required for stability and mobile when mobility is required for movement.

2. *Foot flat (loading response):* Once we've made contact with the ground, the right foot continues to accept our body weight and absorb shock by rolling into pronation. We're shifting our weight into the right leg. We land laterally, roll through the foot into an internally rotated position to set up for the midstance phase. This phase begins when we make initial contact with the right foot and continues until the left foot begins to leave the ground.
3. *Midstance (single-leg stance):* This phase begins when the left foot leaves the ground and continues until the right heel lifts off the ground. We're essentially committing to a single-leg stance and transitioning from a force absorption focus to a forward force propulsion focus. Once here, the heel is now in neutral (not on the lateral end) to center us and get us into a stable,

single-leg stance. The tibia (shin bone) is roughly perpendicular to the floor. The glutes should activate to stabilize the pelvis. The ankle needs around 5 degrees of dorsiflexion to help us with proper mechanics. If ankle mobility is limited, compensations will occur in the walking pattern. Some of the compensation patterns may be walking with the foot in an externally turned-out position (duck walking) or an early heel lift (bouncy gait). If we can't go through a joint in a linear fashion, we'll likely start moving around it. This circumvention decreases overall efficiency and may require us to work harder to propel us forward, because we're no longer moving in straight lines when straight forward motion is required.

4. *Heel off (terminal stance/propulsion):* This phase begins as the right heel leaves the ground and the left foot contacts the ground. As we move through the right foot, we'll start to plantar flex the foot (i.e., the toes flexed or pointing the foot down) and move into hip extension to help propel us forward. The right knee will bend as we toe off. We also want to see sufficient mobility in the big toe joint (first metatarsal joint)—around 60 degrees of extension as you extend the toes when the ball of the foot prepares for push off. Our weight is distributed among the metatarsal heads (big toe pads). We'll also start to see compensations with limited big toe mobility such as an externally turned-out position (duck walk) or a shortened stride. These compensation patterns may limit our ability to propel ourselves forward.
5. *Toe-off (pre-swing):* This phase begins when the left foot contacts the ground and continues until the right foot leaves the ground. This phase is the final element of propulsion as our toes push off the ground.

Swing phase: About 40 percent of our walking time is spent in the swing phase. This time is spent with our right foot off the ground swinging and preparing to land again. Our body is supported by the left leg and foot. When we take two full steps (right and left), about 80 percent of the time will be spent standing on one leg only. The other 20 percent is spent in double support periods where we are transitioning from one foot to the next. Single-leg stability, the ability to land directly over our base of support, hip stability, and ankle-foot mobility are all factors to consider in this phase.

1. *Early swing:* This phase begins when the right foot leaves the ground. We begin to bend the knee and flex the hip forward to prepare for the leg to swing forward.

2. *Midswing:* This phase begins as the right foot flexes to clear the ground and the right leg moves past the left leg. The left shin is vertical, and the right leg will prepare to straighten.
3. *Late swing:* During this phase, the hip is flexed, the knee is straight, and our body shifts forward to prepare for the right heel strike again.

Stride

Step length for many can bc short, especially if the hips are tight and balance is poor. For others, when we want to walk faster, we take bigger steps, thinking this is the best way to walk faster. Stride length may vary depending on speed and purpose. We may need to take larger strides if we're hiking and need to climb over rocks. We may need to take shorter steps if the terrain calls for it. The perfect stride allows you to comfortably land with your center over your base. If you're landing directly over your base of support with good, stacked alignment, the stride length is likely fine. No special formulas are required.

When we're mobile and stable, our strides will feel effortless. Flexibility may limit our optimal stride length. Ryan Grant, certified pedorthist and owner of Solefit, says, "It could be said that the body will walk as efficiently as it can with what it has in terms of strength, mobility, etc. With that being said, it becomes clear as to how important it is to improve 'what we have.' Stride length and cadence are primarily going to be influenced by flexibility and strength limitations. One of the primary limitations on optimal walking technique is the inability to efficiently extend the hip (in large part due to excess sitting). In this case, the best course to improve walking technique would be to spend more time working on increasing flexibility through the hip. It's always so important to look at why we're not walking optimally and fix this first, as opposed to trying to change the way we walk without addressing the cause behind it." You'll find strengthening exercises in chapter 9 and stretches (including hip stretches) in chapter 6.

Walking while carrying a baby, heavy bag, equipment, or other things may cause walking asymmetry. Our steps may not be equal in length, and this may cause discomfort or inequities in weight distribution and load. Walking asymmetry may indicate an injury, spending more time on one leg versus the other when we're in our single-leg stance, or differing step lengths.

Many of us have the technology to evaluate our walking symmetry through our various devices (e.g., phones, watches) and can determine whether adjustments are needed. We're ideally looking for a lower percentage when assessing walking asymmetry. We don't have set numbers as to what is ideal, and many of us will not be perfectly symmetrical between right and left sides, but a percentage higher than 3 to 5 percent may warrant a deeper dive into our gait mechanics.

Land Over Your Foot

When walking, it's important to land with the foot underneath the body. Your center of mass should line up directly over your base of support (our stance limb). Once your foot hits the ground and you've transferred your weight to your stance leg, ideally your body should align. This will ensure effective muscle use. Core and hip muscles fire more efficiently in this stacked position. Landing over your base will also ensure you're moving economically—that is, using the least amount of resources required to propel yourself forward. A well-stacked and positioned system will allow for this. Finally, landing with your center over your base will decrease impact forces. It also works to increase cadence, which also contributes to reduced impact forces. Ardestani et al. (2016) found that individuals who increased cadence but not stride length to walk faster did not experience a significant increase in impact on the joints. Those who increased their stride length or both stride length and cadence experienced a significant increase in all joint impacts. Essentially, those who took bigger steps experienced higher impact on the joints versus those who took smaller, faster steps.

When we take too big of a stride walking, we land with our foot ahead of our bodies, which causes us to overstride (figure 5.2). Overstriding essentially puts the brakes on our systems. Our rhythm gets altered, and that smooth forward moving and circular pattern of the lower body gets jammed in a sense. Overstriding may also lead to low back and other joint discomforts. Gill et al. (2023) found that overstriding predominantly increased peak joint impacts, suggesting that overstriding is more likely to negatively affect injury risk than understriding.

The repetition of joint impacts over time affects the capacity of muscles to withstand and tolerate the increased forces associated with walking with longer strides. This may lead to overuse injuries and discomforts. Strength training and progressively increasing walking volumes and intensities all play a role in increasing the tolerance of our tissues and preventing overuse injuries. However, an easy and intelligent first step is to ensure our stride length is appropriate and efficient. It may seem counterintuitive to take smaller steps, but longer steps may lead to more harm than good when starting out.

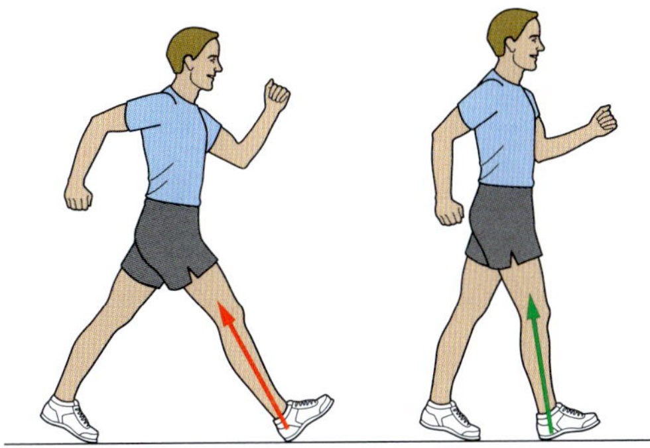

FIGURE 5.2 Overstriding versus landing over base.

Relaxed Walking and Strolling

Not all our walks have to be powerful. When we're walking with friends, out enjoying beautiful weather, traveling and taking in the sights, or taking a family walk after a big meal, these can all be opportunities to move at a slower pace. Time on our feet is beneficial on so many levels, and varying the paces, terrains, and intensities all play a role in overall health. As long as we're including more powerful walks and workouts in our overall plan, the slower, more relaxed walks have an important place in our lives.

We don't have to exaggerate the arm swing on slower walks. It's beneficial to focus on landing with our foot underneath us to ensure we're landing on a stable base. Avoid overstriding, shuffling, or leaning forward at the hips. Maintain good alignment and a stacked ribs-over-hips position to help core muscles engage effortlessly. Once we pick up the pace, we'll want to start thinking about our arm position and swing, stride length, and mechanics a bit more.

Power Walking and Speed Walking

Maybe you've walked with someone who simply could not walk faster (without running). Or maybe you've been that person who simply can't keep up. When we start to pick up speed, our walking mechanics may change a little bit. Our steps should become shorter (at first) and quicker. We'll expand on this in more detail in chapter 7. Overstriding is a common walking pattern that may place additional strain on the lower back, reduce walking efficiency, and alter gait mechanics. Landing with the base of support under the center of mass (i.e., landing with the foot directly under the body) will allow us to absorb, create sufficient ground force, and propel ourselves forward. The short, quick stride will allow us to walk faster and with more efficiency. Try long and short strides and see how you (and your low back) feel. You can work to increase stride length once you've mastered the form.

Start to tighten the arm position when walking at faster speeds (figure 5.3) to prevent slowing down. A long arm lever will create more drag and may place more strain on the shoulder. Tightening the arm position will also help us to walk faster and with more efficiency. Think of runner arms. Close the arm position so that the forearms are close to parallel to the floor. The arm angle will be bent between 45 and 90 degrees. Aim to keep this tight bent-arm position throughout. Try not to straighten and bend your arms as you walk. Keep an aerodynamic, tucked-in arm position and drive your elbows back to help generate more speed and forward motion.

When we want to walk faster, we think of picking up the pace. Shorter steps, tighter arm positions, elbows driving to the back, and pressing the feet into the ground all help to increase our walking speed to more of a power walking pace.

Ankle mobility, thoracic mobility (trunk turning slightly with each step), and pelvis (dissociation and stability) are important to ensure we're walking comfortably and efficiently. Dissociation is the ability to separate segments when required. When we walk, our whole bodies don't move in the same direction. We need a fixed point to move off from. The pelvis and torso are fairly fixed as our arms and legs move off those fixed points. The ability to create fixed points, move from those points, and move only what is required to create forward momentum is key. We land with our foot, it plants into the ground, and we can use that to help us move the other leg forward in just the right amount. Our torso in a sense is fixed so that our opposite arm can swing forward. Without these stable areas and fixed points, we create more unnecessary movement.

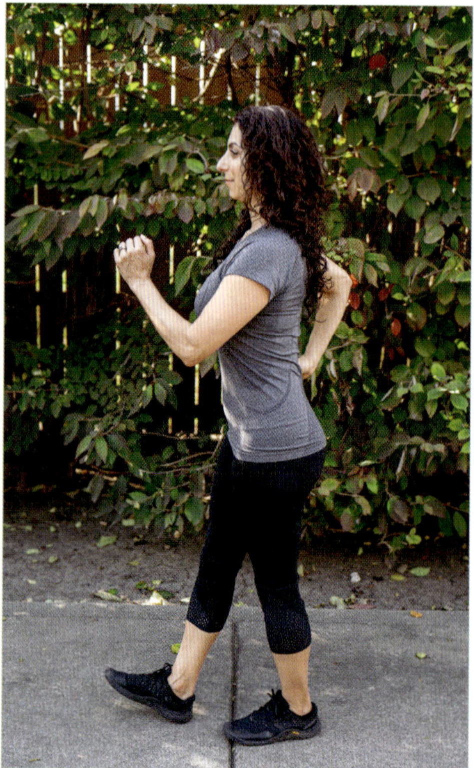

FIGURE 5.3 Tight-arm power walk position.

When walking at faster speeds, we all have a set preferred transition speed at which we would naturally move into a jog or running pattern once we walk at a pace that feels too fast. Studies have shown that walking faster than our preferred transition speed—that is, walking faster, even when we want to break out into a jog—will recruit more muscles, specifically in the quads and calves (Shih et al. 2016). When higher-impact activities like running aren't possible, learning how to walk well and walk faster can boost our overall muscle recruitment.

Race Walking

I can't remember exactly when I tried race walking for the first time, but I do remember how great it felt. I instantly wanted to learn more. It felt challenging, but doable. It was hard to believe you could work so hard while walking! I trained for years with a local race walking club, the Bytown Walkers, and eventually worked up to competing (winning provincial and national races in 2015 in the 5,000 m and 2016 in the 3,000 m, respectively). As a former competitive dancer and international fitness competitor, it was the perfect sport for me at that time. Years of dance and fitness were hard on my system, and race walking was just what I needed to work hard yet be gentle on my body.

The definition of race walking is simple and very specific. Roger Burrows, race walking coach and founder of the Bytown Walkers, explains:

> Race walking is not weird or complicated. It's normal walking tuned up. World Athletics' Book of Rules does not refer to "rules" governing race walking technique. Instead, it refers to a "definition" that describes a "progression of steps" taken in a certain way. Race walking is not seen as an artificial creation but as a simple evolution of the walking, the "progression of steps," that carries us around our world every day. The definition does not tell the world's competitive walkers what to do; it describes what the best of them are already doing. It has two elements, the purpose of which is simply to distinguish walking from running.

The elements are that first, one foot or the other must always be in contact with the ground; second, the advancing leg must be straight at the knee "from the moment of first contact with the ground until the vertical upright position," according to international standards.

"So, race walkers are not seen to be following or breaking 'the rules,' they are seen to be complying or not complying with 'the definition'," shares Burrows.

What do we see when we watch experienced race walkers? Burrows states, "In each phase, we can imagine a snapshot. But the snapshots assembled become, more accurately, frames in a video of what we want to see, and especially, in our own walking, what we want to feel. As we will see later, when the phases become factors in competitive situations, notably race walking, coaches may refer to the video as an athlete's Technical Model."

First, we see a "wheel of feet" where

1. the front foot contacts the ground going backward,
2. it then passes under the body in the vertical position that requires the straight knee, and then
3. the same foot recovers forward close to the ground.

When one leg is at point (3), the other is at point (1) and moves through points (2) and (3) as the first leg carries the foot forward to (1) once more. The whole sequence keeps the wheel of feet rotating at remarkable speeds.

Second, we see a dynamic arm action. As we have discussed, the active arm drive allows us to increase overall walking speeds. "The overall effect is that the body is a big, motionless parcel being carried forward by the arms and legs," shares Burrows.

The curious walker looking to explore race walking can refine normal walking with Burrows' four easy stages:

1. Bend your arms. Walk normally but hold the arms as if you were running.
2. Shorten your stride. As you adapt, your stride will go back to its natural length. Our main goal at this early stage is to increase the rhythm.
3. Use your arms more strongly to help you surge forward. To prepare for the fourth stage, hold on to something secure and stand on one leg. The muscles surrounding the knee should tighten and contract. The knee should also be straight. Try this on both legs. This is the same feeling we are looking to attain in step 4.
4. As you walk with "stage two" quick strides and "stage three" arms, pick one knee and reproduce the muscle contraction you felt when you stood on one foot. After a few repetitions, do the same with the other knee.

Burrows adds, "Don't expect perfectly straight knees to start with. If your knees straighten right away, you are in a lucky minority of natural race walkers. Most of us have to work at it a bit as we start our race walk training. This is because we are asking our muscles—and our brain—to perform an action they have not previously been used to. We include basic 'skill' exercises in our warm-ups or training sessions, just like accomplished musicians practice their basic skills before a performance or rehearsal." There are several race walking clubs across Canada and the United States. I would encourage anyone interested to reach out to your local clubs.

Burrows concludes by asking us all to counter some misinformation often heard about race walking:

> Even in the highest level of competition, the unbroken contact with the ground is *as seen by the unaided eye*. Photographs or slow-motion videos showing loss of contact as alleged evidence of an infraction actually mean nothing unless the experienced judges on site see it too (and three of them have to independently agree). Two factors provide the explanation. First, the human eye records motion at a slower rate than a camera. Second, and more important, video doesn't tell us anything walkers don't already know: Fast walking of any kind has a brief period of "flight" on every step. A slo-mo video would likely show us breaking contact when we hurry for the bus!

Walking Strategies (Feet, Arms, Legs)

While walking, we are imposing an impact force of between 1 and 1.5 times our bodyweight. Our body absorbs these forces, stores them, and we release almost double of that upon release. We essentially double the amount of energy coming in via absorption and recoil mechanics. This is mostly done through our fascial system. Our fascia can store and return energy, and this system is key for our bodies to experience elastic recoil. Human fascia has a high energy return capacity, which is key for movement efficiency. The potential energy turns into elastic energy via our tendons and fascia. There's an elastic recoil element in dynamic movement just as there is in a spring (think of a gazelle's spring-like movement). Studies have found that human fascia has energy storage capacity similar to kangaroos and gazelles (Sawicki et al. 2009). Walking is more of a fascial response. The more of this elastic recoil we can harness, the less effort is required to move. Tendons can recoil elastically much faster than muscles can shorten (Alexander 2002). We don't want to muscle through our movements; we want to absorb impact forces and release them with efficiency via the elastic recoil of fascia. If we're moving with muscles, it's not very efficient. Moving fascially is economical.

Dr. Emily Splichal, functional podiatrist and founder and CEO of Naboso, explains:

> With every step we take we experience ground reaction forces, forces that become our body's potential energy to take the next step. This relationship with the ground and impact forces is optimal in movement efficiency and movement longevity. This relationship starts with perception, or the awareness of the ground reaction forces.

> The nerves in our feet perceive ground reaction forces as vibration. Cushion in shoes, socks, and arch supports can interfere with our foot's ability to feel these vibrations, making us disconnected from our movement. Upon perceiving these vibrations, the muscles in our feet contract, which dampens the impact and allows the body to store this potential energy in the fascia or connective tissues. Referred to as the Muscle Tuning Theory, muscle contractions dampening vibrations is a critical part of human movement and one that is often overlooked in orthopedics and sports medicine. Upon taking our next step, the potential energy of the ground reaction forces is released from our fascia as elastic energy. This elastic energy transfer is the basis of movement efficiency.

We ideally want to rely on our fascia and on energy coming in from impact forces, absorbing it, storing it, and releasing or recoiling it. We allow this to happen with proper positioning; alignment; stacking; breathing; muscle firing, patterning, and connecting; timing; and good proprioceptive awareness.

Starting with a good foot-to-ground connection will help us feel the ground, create a solid fixed point, and improve proprioceptive awareness and core connections. According to Dr. Splichal, "When we walk, the initial contact of the foot is on the outside, lateral aspect of our heel. There is an important functional reason for this foot position during walking. First, this places the foot in a stable or inverted position, which prepares the foot to unlock or evert in order to absorb impact forces. If the foot position upon contact is not stable then the ability to absorb impact forces is more difficult and can increase the risk of impact-related injuries such as plantar fasciitis, shin splints, or stress fractures." During your warm-up, think about feeling the foot connecting to the ground. This strong connection allows us to work up the chain to help create good stability, mobility, and forward propulsion.

We also want to ensure we're using our arms and legs efficiently with the (possibly shorter) stride. A tight arm swing with faster walking paces allows us to walk efficiently, and the backward arm drive creates forward momentum. Think of driving the arm backward (and not forward) to create forward momentum. Just as a slingshot begins by pulling back, the backward arm drive helps to propel us forward. Our legs will create a solid pillar or single-leg stance as we move through the various phases of gait. We also want to spend equal amounts of time on each leg. Our watches, phones, and other devices may help us to identify potential walking asymmetries. We want to walk with optimal alignment and breathing, as covered in chapter 4. As we pick up the pace, we want to avoid compensating. After addressing walking speed, we discuss some of the more common walking patterns to avoid.

Walking Mechanics Tips

Good walking mechanics involve

1. Balance and stability on one leg;
2. Optimal stacking of the body;
3. On impact, the ability to absorb impact forces through fascia, muscles, and proprioception;
4. Optimal stride mechanics; and
5. Forward motion.

Walking Speed

Although it's not necessary for all our walks to be fast, we ideally don't want all of our walks to be slow. In older adults, slow gait speeds may be a predictor of mortality and cardiovascular disease. A 2018 meta-analysis found that each reduction of 0.1 meters per second in gait speed was associated with a 12 percent increased risk of earlier mortality and an 8 percent increased risk of cardiovascular disease (Veronese et al. 2018). Del Pozo Cruz et al. (2022) found that there are greater health benefits to walking faster. In this study, those who walked 80 steps per minute reduced their risk of cardiovascular disease, cancer, and premature death compared to those walking 40 steps per minute (which would be described as a typical pace for those moving place to place). Further, those who walked even faster at 112 steps per minute reduced their risk of dementia by 38 percent.

When heading out the door for a walk, spend a moment to set an intention for your walk, and if possible, aim to have most of your walks be at moderate or faster speeds and intensities.

Walking Patterns to Avoid

A handful of walking patterns should ideally be avoided. They may be inefficient and cause pain or discomfort, and they may be hard to identify by feel. Having someone take a video of you walking may be helpful in identifying any potential ineffective walking patterns. There are many who walk and walk quickly and comfortably with these walking patterns; however, identifying and changing them may help to increase walking speed and comfort even more.

Windshield Wipers

When our posture tends to be a bit more rounded and shoulders are turned inward (internally rotated), the arms may cross the midline of the body during arm swing. Aim to keep your arms in front of you without having them cross the middle of the body. This cross-body action may slow us down, reinforce the internally rotated shoulder position (or not help it), and may load the front of the shoulders excessively. Keep the arms by your sides in a smooth forward and back motion. Regarding your arms, find your lane and stay in your lane.

Hands/Wrists Coming Up Too High

An excessive arm swing may bring the arms up too high, placing additional strain on the shoulders. If the arms are bent, ideally the thumbs should come up to chest height at the top of arm swing, no higher, and to the hip (around the iliac crest) at the bottom of the arm swing, no farther.

Leaning Forward at the Hips

Leaning too far forward at the waist or hip area places additional load on the lower back and will inevitably slow us down and decrease our overall walking economy. Aim to bend from the ankles if at all and keep the waist or hip line smooth to ensure a solid hip extension pattern.

Lumbering

When overall single-leg stability is decreased, we may widen our stance and move in a more side-to-side motion in which the head comes up, over, and down to one side instead of remaining fairly level. We don't necessarily want to be walking on a tightrope line, but we also don't want to be walking on a train track line. Include some single-leg balance work, aim to tighten the walking line slightly, and slow the gait down to determine where the breaks in the pattern are occurring.

Overstriding

This is a tricky one. When we want to walk faster, we think taking bigger steps will accomplish this. This only works if you're able to land with your center of mass directly over your base of support, but this is challenging with large strides. For most people, taking smaller, quicker steps allows us to properly absorb and respond to ground forces and effectively propel ourselves forward without placing additional strain on our backs or joints.

Shuffling

As we age, this pattern becomes more evident as our overall stability and balance are reduced. A shuffling walking pattern decreases overall efficiency. If stability is lacking, walking with poles may be an alternative to help with proper foot striking, roll through, and push off.

Essentially, we want to improve efficiency, and some of these walking patterns decrease overall walking efficiency. We want to limit landing too heavy, being too bouncy, taking steps that are too big or too small, and using our arms in a way that doesn't support and propel us forward. The body ideally should face in the direction it's moving. Our feet, arms, and hands all guide us to the direction in which we're heading. We want forward motion, not upward or sideway motion. Although limb length, environment, history, balance, stability, and goals will dictate the way we walk, we ideally want to walk with efficiency and increased comfort.

Walking With Children and Dogs

Our gait will likely change when we're walking and pushing a stroller, carrying or holding our children, or walking with our dogs. Although it can be challenging to focus on making changes to our gait while we're holding a wiggly toddler, we've included some tips and strategies to help mitigate potential discomforts.

Walking With a Dog

Walking a dog on a leash can alter gait mechanics and potentially lead to discomforts or repetitive injuries. Even with a well-trained dog who walks loosely on a leash, I still find my gait is not the same as without. For healthy people who have higher capacities in general, it's likely not a big issue, but individuals with lower thresholds and dogs that pull more aggressively might experience discomfort or repetitive strain.

It also depends on how hard a dog is pulling. Light pulling can lead to smaller shifts, and in healthy individuals who can tolerate the load and who have higher capacities in general, it may be a minor detail. Someone with lower thresholds and a dog that pulls quite aggressively may start to experience discomfort. If you're a dog walker and notice that your shoulders, back, or hips experience pain, take a closer look at the mechanics of your gait. Are there strategies or tools to make your dog pull less? It's no easy feat! I spent months training our puppy to loose-leash walk (in the winter!), because I remember the challenges of having a dog that pulls. Even in strong walkers, the pulling can lead to mild discomforts.

From a mechanical perspective, the leash prevents you from fully driving the arm or elbow back. The backward arm drive allows for more forward momentum. This shift will lead to asymmetries as well as potential shifts in speed, velocity, or intensity. If you consistently hold the leash in one hand, it can create an asymmetrical pattern in your gait. This asymmetry may affect your body's alignment, potentially impacting the muscles and joints on one side of your body more than the other. A waist leash may serve as a possible alternative; however, you will likely still be pulled to one side.

Dog pulling is going to add rotational forces, causing more thoracic and possibly lumbo-pelvic rotation to one side. This additional rotational force may challenge the pelvis and thoracic spine. Many individuals complain of one-sided shoulder, back, sacroiliac, and pelvic pain when being pulled by a dog. (We love them though, don't we?) Also, from an asymmetrical perspective, the pulling may cause the walker to spend more time on one leg versus the other. The timing should be equitable right to left, and a longer one-sided load may cause potential issues. Again, for most of us, walking our dogs is a pleasant and energizing outing. If you're noticing discomforts, it might be worth exploring further.

Dog Walking Tips

1. Encourage less pulling when possible.
2. Use tools such as harnesses to lessen pulling.
3. Alternate leash walking hand.
4. Observe gait and adjust as needed.
5. Seek help at the onset of pain.

Walking With a Stroller

Many new parents will spend years walking and pushing their child(ren) in a stroller. It's a great opportunity for parents to get outside and integrate movement in the day, and our children enjoy the fresh air and taking in the sights. Pushing an object in front of us with both hands limits our ability to use our arms, limits our thoracic rotation, and alters our mechanics. As our children get older and heavier, the load becomes more challenging to push. We ideally want to keep our spines straight and avoid leaning forward at the waist. Maintaining an upright posture will allow us to use our hips more effectively and decrease the load on our lumbar spines and surrounding musculature.

To allow a more fluid and rhythmic walking pattern, aim to use one hand or arm to push the stroller, placing the hand closer to the center to keep the stroller centered. The other arm can then swing naturally, allowing our spine and pelvis to move freely. As a mother of two children, I remember this was not easy! There were years of walking while pushing various strollers or holding my child in a carrier (front and back) or in my arms when they became too tired to walk. For many new parents, focusing on walking form and technique may be the last thing on your minds. If you're a new parent experiencing pain or discomfort, straightening the spine and alternating the hand on the stroller may be helpful.

We've covered the various parts of walking mechanics, and now we want to put it all together in a way that feels right for us. Not every walk needs to be intense or purposeful. My daily walks include faster-paced walks, racing walks, slower walks, and leisurely strolls. They all play a part in my overall walking program that includes elements of fitness, sociability, nature, and joy.

PART III

PREPARE FOR YOUR WORKOUT

CHAPTER 6

Warm Up and Cool Down

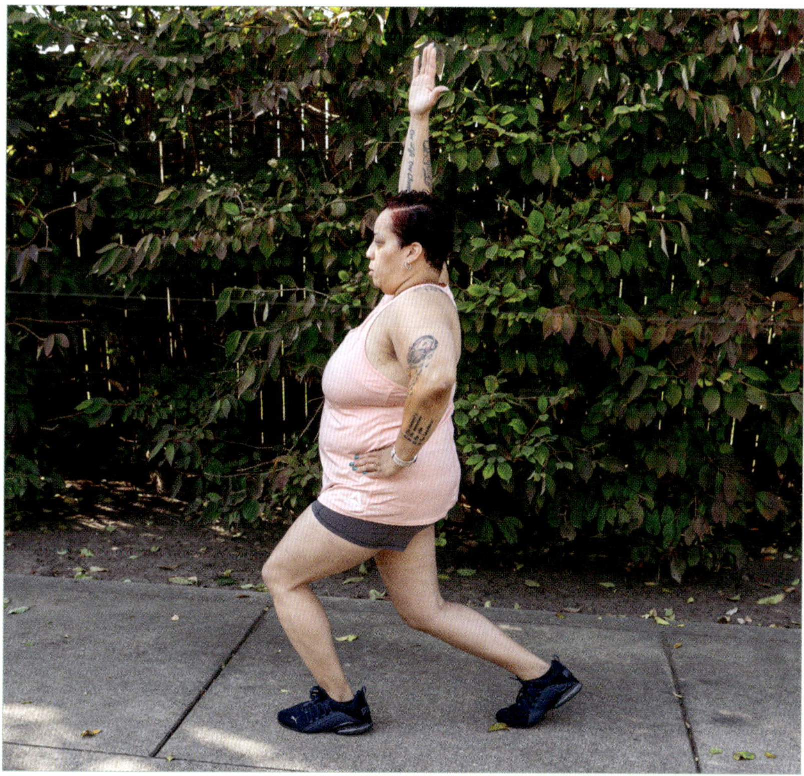

You're dressed, ready to go, and keen to hit the road. You get out there and jump right into your walking pace. I've been there! Ensuring we are well warmed up helps prepare our bodies for walking, allows our cardiovascular systems a chance to slowly ramp up, and gives our muscles a chance to get prepped and primed, ready for what's to come. Taking a few minutes to prepare our bodies for our walks helps us work at our best.

Taking some time to prepare for your activity can make a big difference in how you feel. Roger Burrows, race walking coach and founder of the Bytown Walkers, describes the warm-up as "a period of transition from daily activity to the exercise activity. The transition is a physical and mental rehearsal, with both aspects combining into a process of 'getting in the mood.' Performers of all kinds (athletes, actors, musicians) all have a process that prepares them specifically for the activity to follow. Athletes in skill-based events are particularly careful about planning their warm-up accordingly. I have used the image of driving up a ramp onto a freeway." When I'm properly warmed up, physical activity feels easier and gentler, and I feel better prepared to push a bit harder.

Research has shown that warming up prior to exercise can improve overall performance (Fradkin et al. 2010; McGowan et al. 2015). Depending on the type of exerciser you are, you may want to head out the door and start with an easy walk to warm up. For many, that can be an effective way to prepare for your walk. Walking and easing into your desired pace is a good way to warm up and ensure your body is prepared for your subsequent walking workout.

For others, taking a bit more time to actively and dynamically warm up, prepare your muscles and tissues for your activity, and create an ideal environment to push a bit harder might be best. Our bodies and brains need an adjustment period and time to bridge the gap. The warm-up is important for our bodies and for our brains as we cement ideal patterns, signals, and pathways that allow us to move with ease. As we age, taking a bit more time to prepare might be warranted. As I approach the half-century mark, my body appreciates a few extra minutes of priming before movement, especially before higher-intensity workouts. Things just feel better generally for me if I'm well warmed up. (I've learned this the hard way over the years.)

Specific warm-ups might be particularly helpful for those coming off an injury, starting something new, or for those working at higher intensities. Taking time to include dynamic warm-ups followed by some key corrective exercises allows me to perform at my best. If you've had a back injury and you've been prescribed back-specific movements, including some of your back rehabilitation exercises in your warm-up might be helpful. If you tend to feel discomfort in your hips when walking, adding a bit of extra hip mobility and stability before your walk might help alleviate that discomfort. If your heel is what tends to feel achy first, dynamic calf stretches followed by hip activation might do the trick. Although getting assessed by a professional will allow you to tailor your corrective exercises, these general tips might be helpful.

In this chapter, we've outlined some specific, purposeful, dynamic warm-up drills that can be included on your subsequent walks. After walking for a few minutes, aim to perform a few repetitions of each of the following drills, or at least a handful of them if you're short on time. Alternatively, you can pick the drills that are most relevant to you and the body parts that need the most attention. There should be no pain or discomfort with any of the movements. If you feel discomfort, aim to modify or omit the activity.

Walking as a Warm-Up

It is appropriate to ease into your walking workout at a slower pace, especially if you're walking at lower and moderate intensities. Begin with 3 to 5 minutes of a slightly slower pace and gradually increase your walking speed to your desired pace. I will often solely use this as my warm-up for slow- to moderate-paced walks.

Suggested Workout Order With Warm-Up and Cool-Down

1. Walking warm-up: 3 to 5 minutes
2. Dynamic purposeful warm-up drills: 2 to 5 minutes
3. Walking workout: the main event
4. Cool-down: 3 to 5 minutes
5. Static stretches: 3 to 5 minutes or longer, if desired

Dynamic Warm-Ups

These dynamic warm-up drills are purposeful and specific to help prepare you for more intense walks. They are appropriate for any level of walking and beneficial to include if you're someone who needs a bit more time getting your tissues primed for your workouts. Perform three to five repetitions of your chosen drill. Beginning with a few minutes at a slower pace first to increase blood flow is a good lead up to these dynamic warm-up drills.

ANKLE ROTATIONS

This can be a great start to your active warm-ups right at your chair or desk. Warming up the ankles can be helpful in mobilizing the tissues and joints and creating awareness of and bringing comfort to this area.

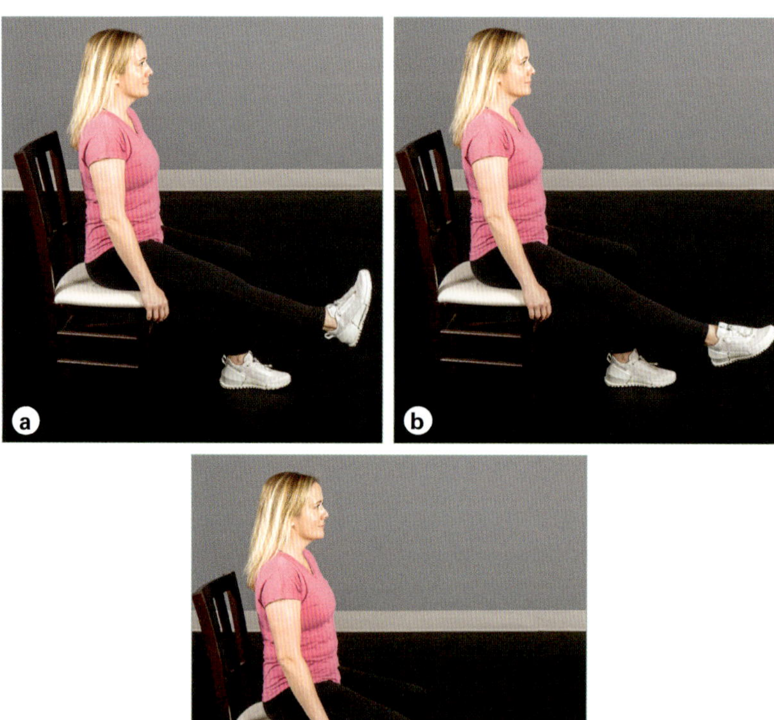

Instructions

From a standing or seated position, create a circle with your foot in one direction and switch to the other direction, then switch feet *(a-c)*. Circle your ankle slowly and aim to move through your full range of motion. Repeat with the other ankle.

Variations

The ankle circles can be done in a supine position, lying on your back with your leg extended. For a balance challenge, perform the ankle circles in a standing position or hold on to a wall or secure object for more stability. The ankle movement can also be performed by tracing alphabets instead of only circles for a more multiplanar emphasis.

STANDING CAT/COW

The cat/cow (in any variation) is typically where I start warming up, and it is key to keeping my back feeling comfortable. An effective segmental mobilizer of the spine, the cat/cow is a great movement to identify tight zones, move through an active full range of motion, and stretch several muscles along the back.

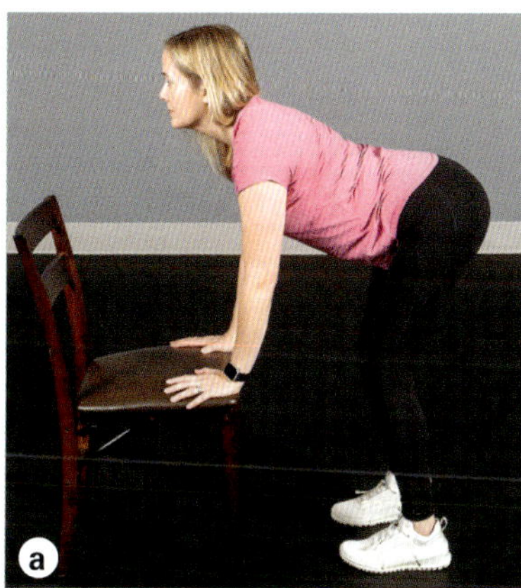
a

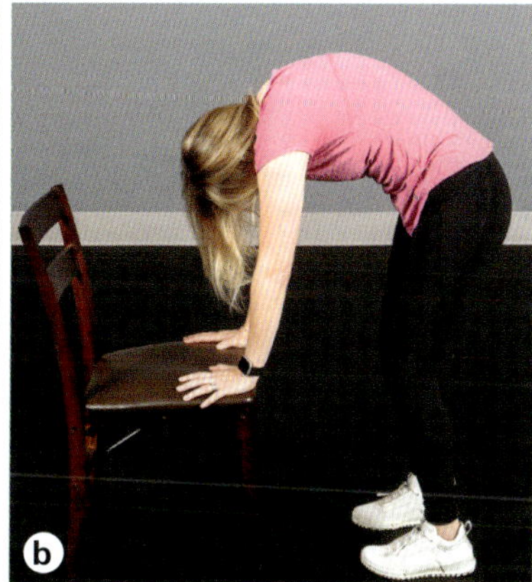
b

Instructions

Begin by standing with your hands at the end of a chair. Knees are soft, shoulders are directly over your wrists, and hips are over your ankles. Inhale to puff your chest out, gently look up, and arch your back *(a)*. Exhale to tuck your chin and tailbone in, and round your back and shoulders *(b)*.

Variations

The cat/cow can also be performed while seated in a chair. Begin seated at the edge of your chair. Place your hands on your thighs and sit tall with good posture. Inhale to puff your chest out, gently look up, and arch your back *(c)*. Exhale to tuck your chin in and round your back and shoulders *(d)*.

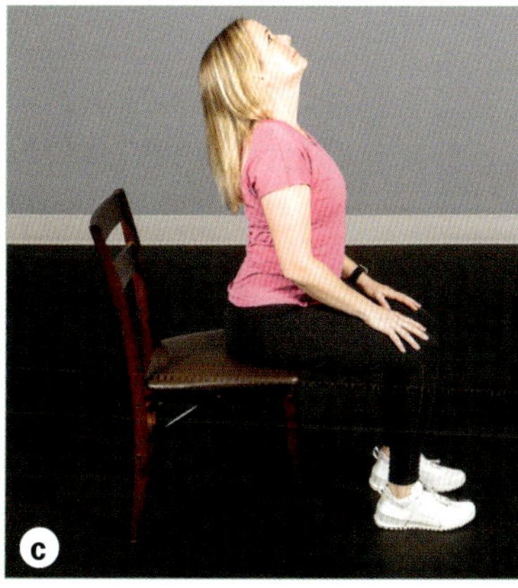
c

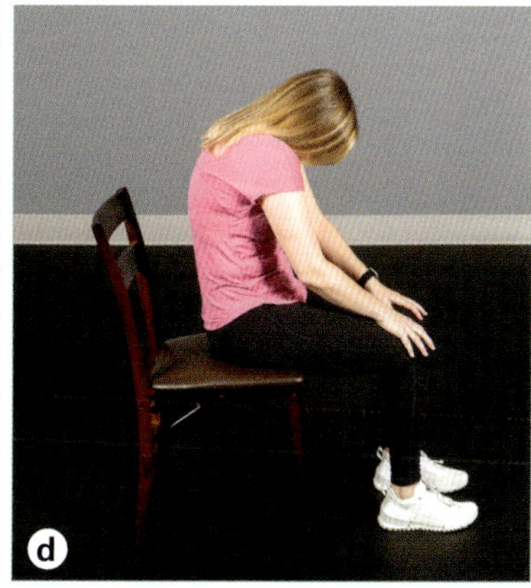
d

Alternatively, the cat/cow can be performed in a quadruped or all-four's position with the hands and knees on the floor *(e-f)*. You can explore rocking back slightly on the cat or cow to feel a deeper stretch in the back *(g)*. Try moving the hips back slightly and performing the cat/cow with a lumbar bias or dropping to the forearms to bias the thoracic spine.

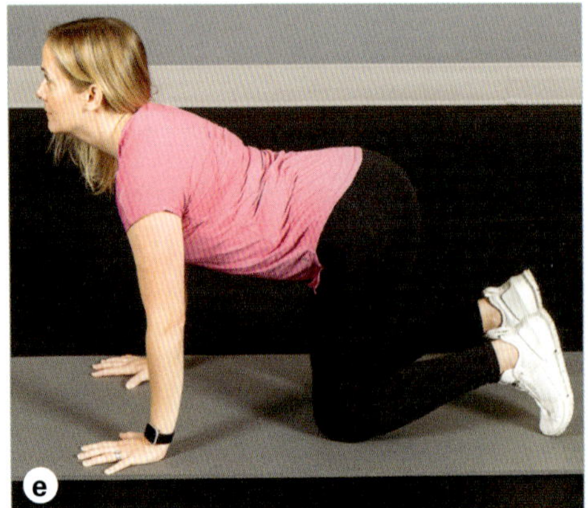
e

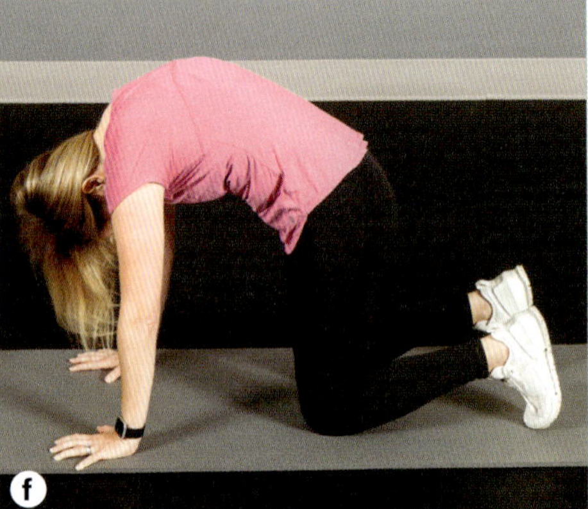
f

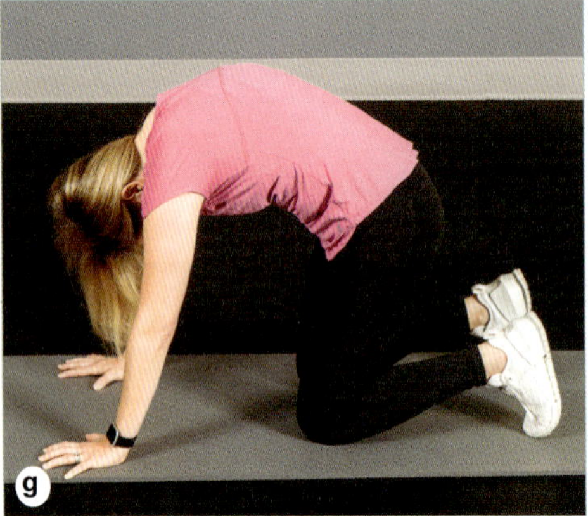
g

BABY STEPS

When I first started race walking competitively, Coach Roger Burrows would guide us through a skill specific warm-up. One of his preferred walking drills is baby steps. “Just 3 to 5 reps of 60 m or so, shortening the stride to half its regular length, and doubling the rhythm as a result.” We’ll further discuss the importance of short strides in chapter 7, and the baby steps drill encourages this quick rhythm with short strides.

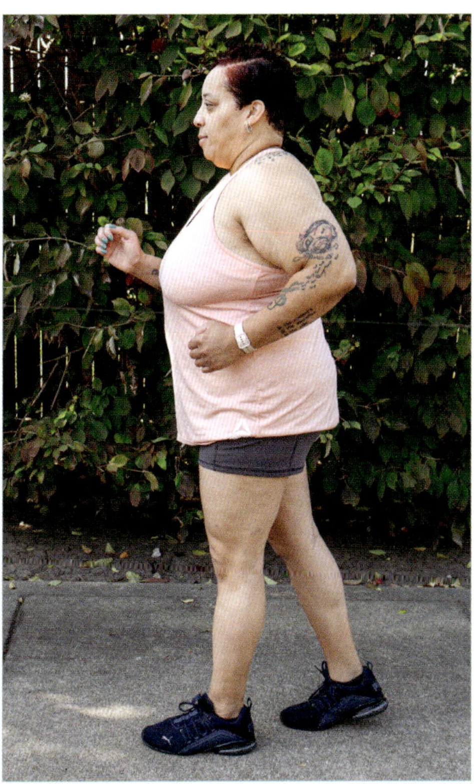

Instructions

Begin by walking slowly with short strides (about half of your regular stride length), aiming to flex the ankle and bend the knees.

Variation

Quicken the pace yet keep the strides short.

HEEL AND TOE WALK

This drill provides an opportunity to eccentrically load the calves and shins, allowing us to build a bit of strength, warm up the lower leg muscles, and bring about some awareness to these key areas.

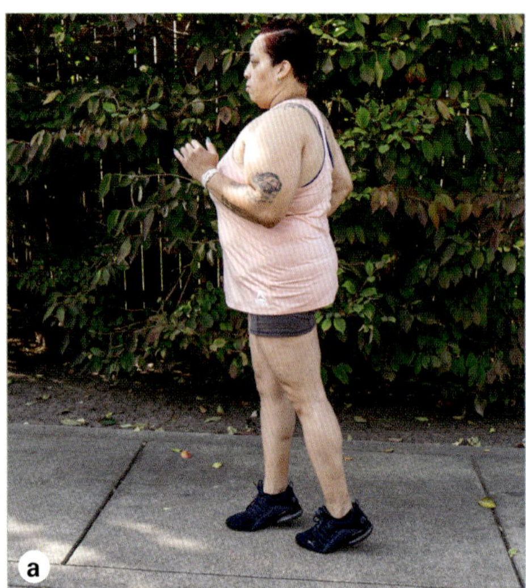
a

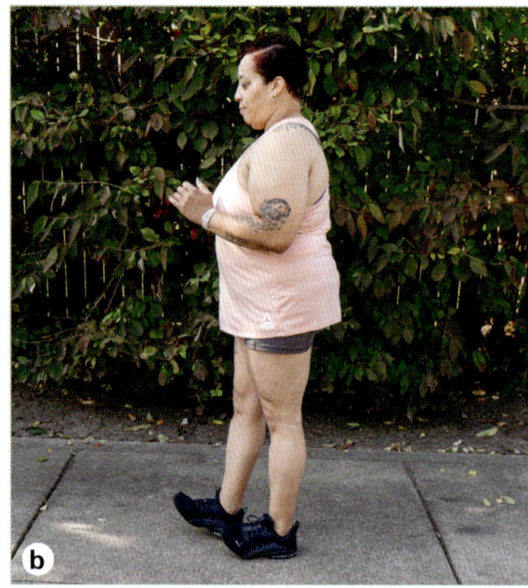
b

Instructions

Take a few steps walking high on the balls of your feet *(a)*, then take a few steps walking on the heels with the toes lifted if balance allows *(b)*.

Variations

Turning the foot in or out slightly will focus on slightly different vectors of the muscles. A turned-in position will focus more on the medial (inner) aspect of the calves, and a turned-out position will focus more on the lateral (outer) aspect of the calves.

WALKING KNEE TO CHEST

The walking knee to chest can prime the single-leg stability and linear pattern of walking as well as include a bit of lumbar flexion and stretch to the low back. It is a great active stretch to help improve balance and stability. It will activate the hip flexors of the bent knee and the hip extensors of the stance leg.

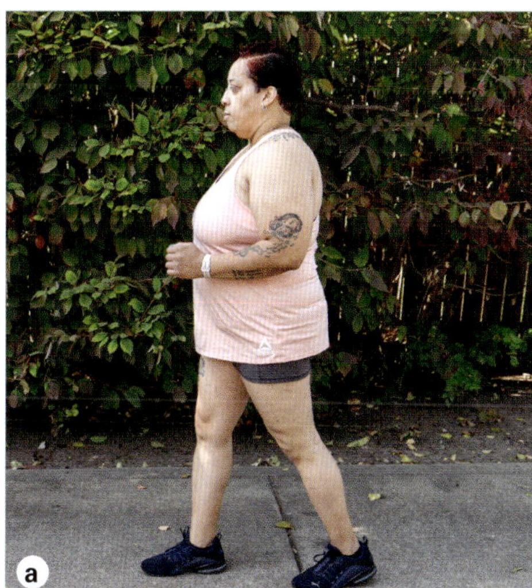
a

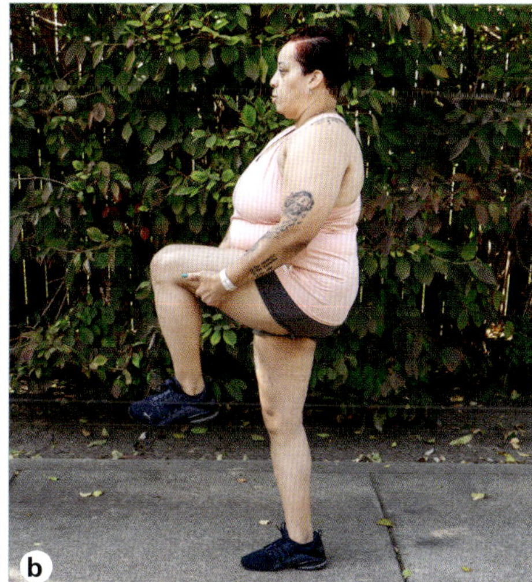
b

Instructions

Begin by standing tall with good posture. Take a step forward with your right leg *(a)* and bring your left leg up toward your chest, holding on to the back of your thigh or front of your shin *(b)*. Bring the left leg back to the ground, then take a step with your left leg and bring your right leg up, holding in the same manner. If you're unable to reach your leg, you can bend your knee and bring it up toward the chest without holding it.

Variations

This drill can also be performed seated or lying on your back. From a seated position, bring your knee up toward your chest, either holding on to the back of your thigh *(c)* or slowly alternating a marching pattern. Alternatively, you can lie on your back and bring one bent leg toward your chest *(d)*. Slowly switch sides.

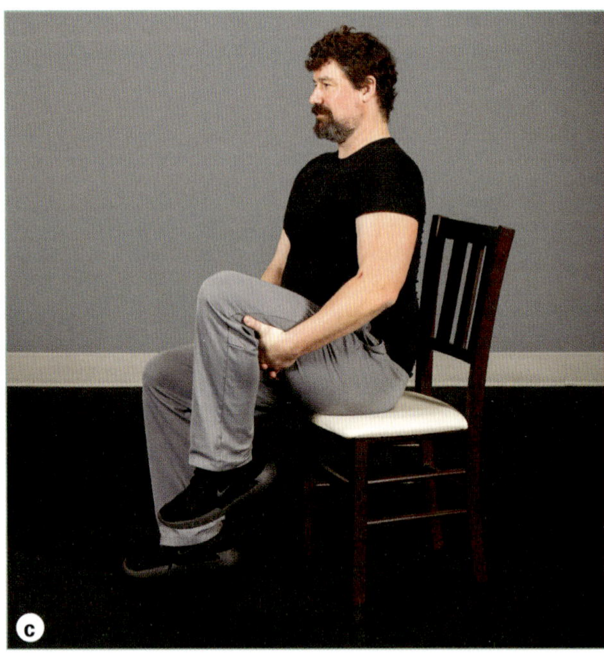

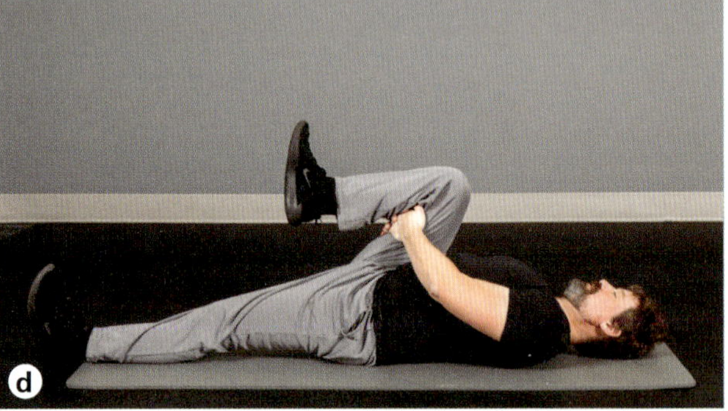

WALKING HIP FLEXOR STRETCH

Although many of us have hip flexors that are weak, they may also be tight. Opening this area can feel great, especially for those who are seated for long periods of time.

Instructions

Take a step forward with your right leg and pause, keeping your left toes on the floor. Bend both knees slightly and perform a pelvic tilt—that is, tuck your pelvis under into a posterior pelvic tilt (if your pelvis was like a bucket filled with water, the water would pour out backward). Aim to tuck the pelvis to lengthen the front of the hip of the back leg *(a)*. Pause in this stretch for a second or two before taking another step to switch sides. Continue walking forward, focusing on the hip flexors and alternating sides.

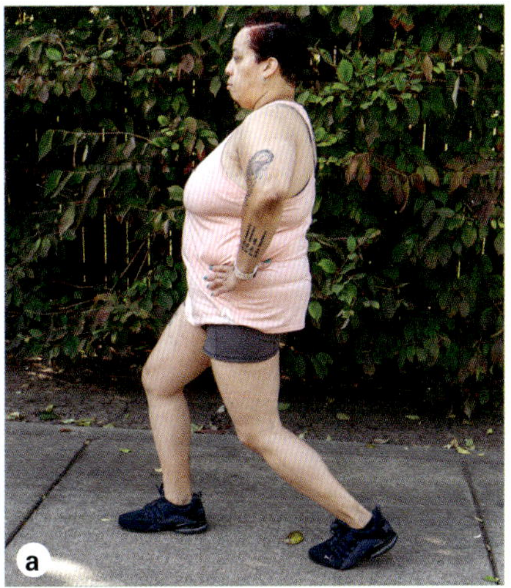
a

Variations

For a more intense stretch, reach one *(b)* or both arms *(c)* up overhead during the pelvic tilt. Whichever leg is back, that is the arm going up if raising one arm. Play around with the angles to find your best stretch. You can reach the arm up and over slightly to target slightly different areas. For an easier variation, perform this drill holding on to a wall, bench, or stable object.

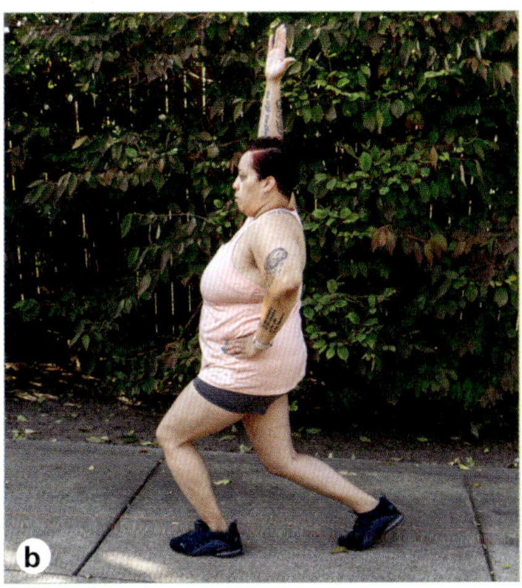
b

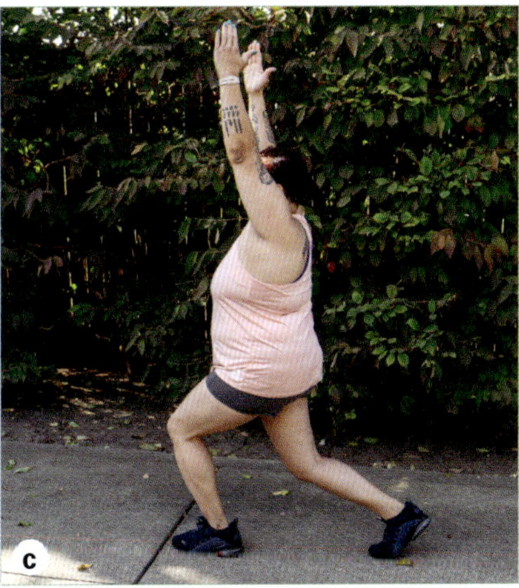
c

DYNAMIC WALKING SHIN STRETCH

Many walkers experience tight and sore shins. I've played around with several variations, but this shin stretch, along with the standing shin stretch cross over (see "Static Stretches"), seem to be the most effective. You can include these dynamic stretches before walking and then repeat them with a static hold after walking.

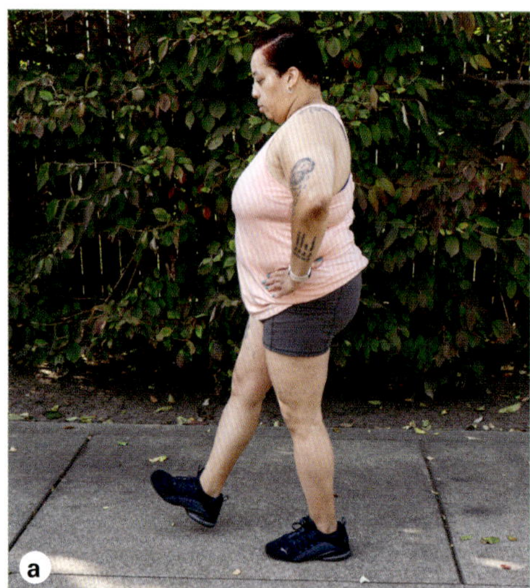

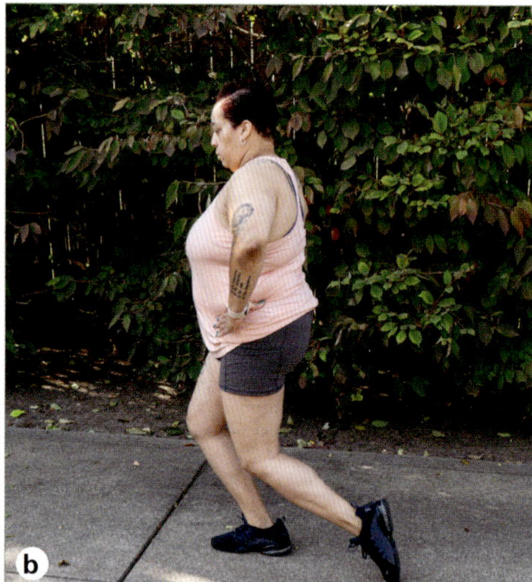

Instructions

Take a step forward with your right leg *(a)*, pause, and turn the top of your left foot down so that your left shoelaces face the floor. Bend both knees and gently press the top of the left foot toward the floor to feel a stretch in the tibialis anterior or shin area *(b)*. Step forward with the left foot and repeat on the right side.

Variations

A deeper knee bend or slightly longer pause will help to intensify the stretch. Holding on to a wall, railing, or stable object will provide more stability.

DUCK WALK

For those with tight calves and Achilles tendons, the duck walk can help to bring some awareness and mobility to these areas. Move slowly and pause in zones that feel tight or restricted.

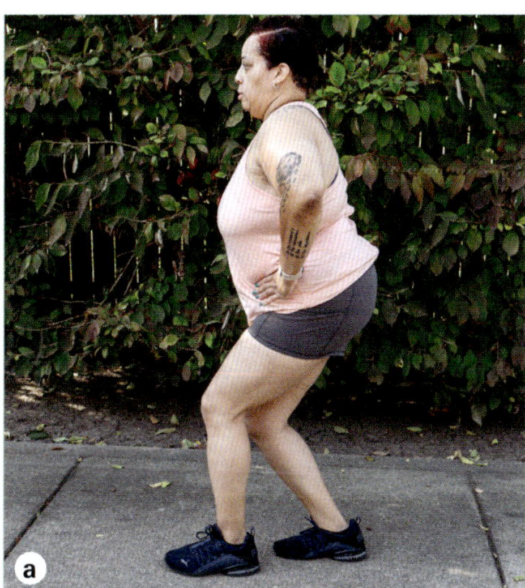

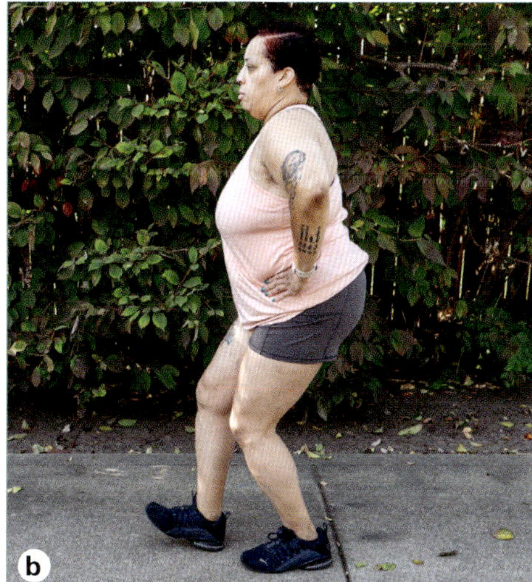

Instructions

Begin by taking slow, small steps. On each step, bend both knees to feel a stretch in the Achilles area (back of the ankle) and calf *(a-b)*. Bend the knees as much as you're comfortable and roll through the foot on each step.

Variations

Bending lower into the knee bend might provide a deeper stretch. Alternatively, you can perform two or three duck walks, take a break with a few regular walking steps, and repeat to break up the movement.

SHOULDER ROLLS AND ARM ROLLS

Many of us hold tension in the neck and shoulders, and simply adding some rolls and movement can help to release tension, bring about some awareness, and relieve stress. Work on breathing through these motions. Circling forward can be an option; however, many of us are stuck in forward rounded-shoulder positions, so I prefer circling backward to help correct and encourage optimal shoulder positioning.

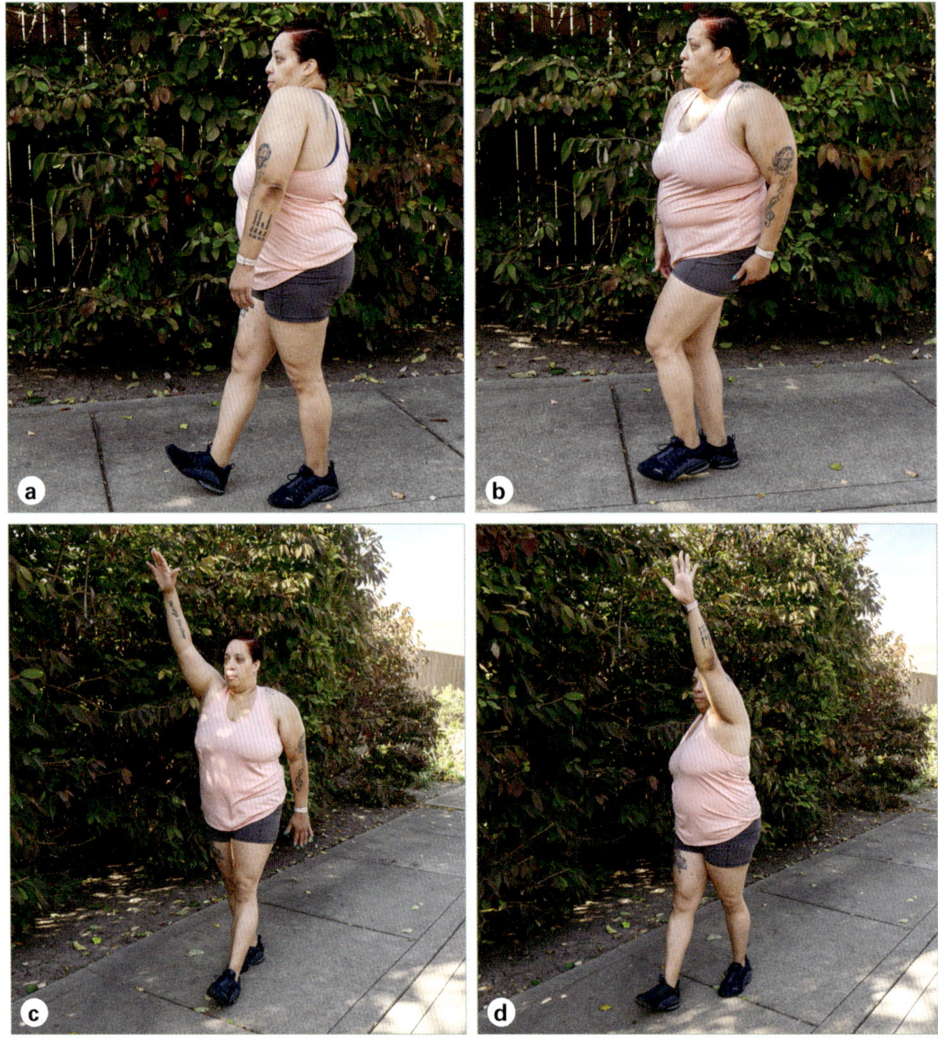

Instructions

Begin by walking slowly. As you take a step forward, circle one shoulder up and back in a circular motion *(a)*. Switch shoulders as you step forward with the other leg *(b)*. After a few shoulder rolls, begin circling the whole arm backward *(c-d)*. You can circle the opposite or same-side arm with the forward step. Move in a way that is comfortable for you.

Variations

If alternating sides is a bit tricky, try circling both shoulders up and back with every second step forward. The arm circles can be spaced out to every second or third step for an easier variation.

WALKING HAMSTRING STRETCH

The walking hamstring stretch will help to provide a stretch to the back of the legs in the hamstrings. Adding a sweeping motion with the arms creates a nice flow of movement.

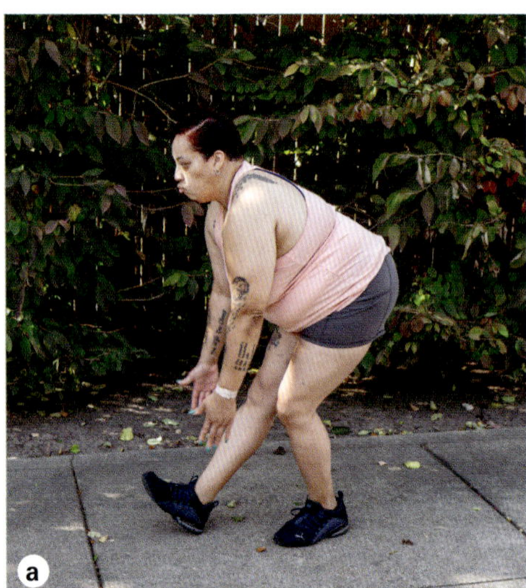
a

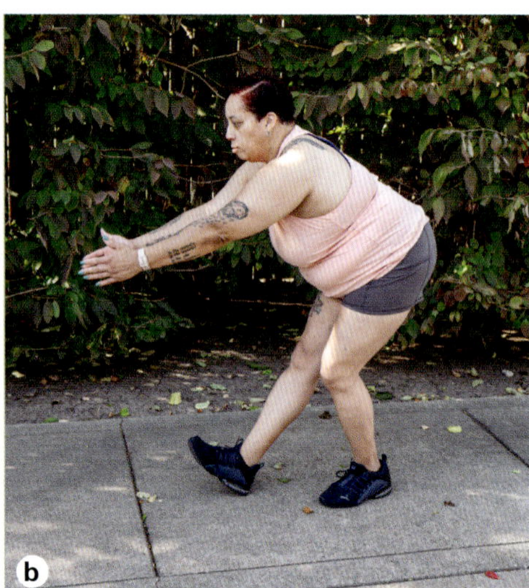
b

Instructions

Begin by standing tall and extend one leg forward. Straighten the leg and lean forward with a straight back, thinking of moving your sit bones to the ceiling or sky behind you *(a)*. Place your hands on your hips or reach forward. Lean forward with a straight back until you feel a gentle hamstring stretch *(b)*. Take two regular steps and repeat the stretch on the other side.

Variation

If leaning forward is uncomfortable, try taking a step and lifting the other leg straight up. Aim to lift the leg comfortably until you feel a gentle stretch in the hamstring (*c-d*). Continue stepping and kicking forward with a slight bend in the kicking leg. Stay within a comfortable range.

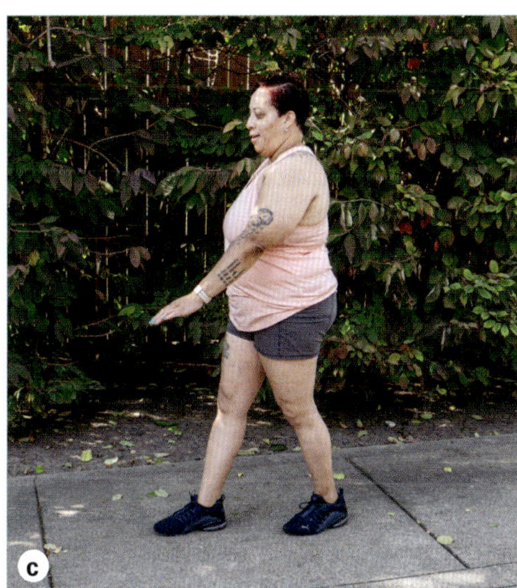
c

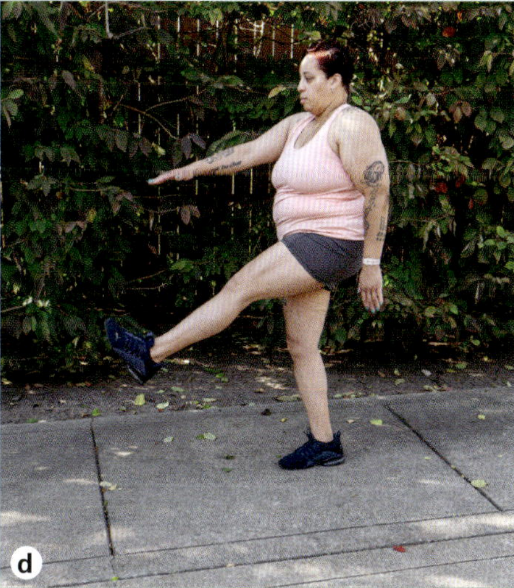
d

Cool-Down

Spending a few minutes (or longer) decreasing your overall pace is an important element of cooling down. A slower walk, especially after a more vigorous walk, can help with recovery, comfort, and a gentle easing back to homeostasis. This allows our cardiovascular system indicators like blood pressure and heart rate to gradually lower to resting levels. It gives us a chance to catch our breath and provides a sense of overall integration of the work we've done. Although we don't have strong evidence surrounding active cool-downs and muscular recovery and recuperation, I find it helpful to spend a few minutes slowing down before stretching while our tissues are warm (Van Hooren and Peake 2018).

Try the following stretches and select the ones that feel best for you. Pick a handful, ideally stretching the areas in the major muscle groups with some extra focus on muscles that feel tight or restricted for you. Breathe during the stretches; avoid holding your breath. Particularly if your shins are tight or sore during or after faster walks, include these in your postwalk stretches. Hold each stretch for 15 to 60 seconds, depending on comfort and your specific goals.

STANDING QUAD STRETCH

For some, this is an uncomfortable stretch, and I recommend using the variation that feels best for you. The quad stretch is effective at stretching the front of the leg. Adding this stretch after a walk when the muscles are warm is effective at improving range of motion and comfort in this area.

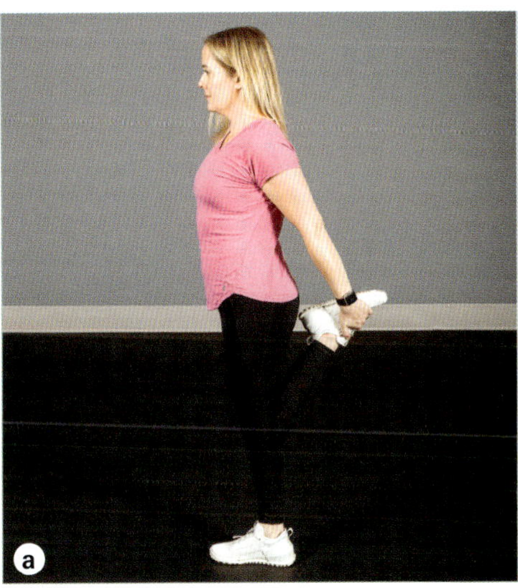

Instructions

Begin by standing tall with one hand against something stable (e.g., wall, tree, bench, car). Bend one leg and reach that same arm behind you to hold on to the ankle or foot. Bring your knees side by side, if possible, bend your standing leg slightly, and gently push your hips forward *(a)*. If grabbing the ankle is not within your accessible range of motion, you can place your leg behind you on a bench, chair, couch, and so on and push your hips forward while keeping your knees side by side. Hold for time, and switch to the other side.

Variations

The quad stretch can be performed in a side-lying position. Lie on your side with your bottom arm supporting your head. Bend your top leg and reach for your ankle or foot *(b)*. This stretch can also be done lying prone on your stomach. With your head down, reach back for your ankle or foot and hold *(c)*. If necessary, use a strap or towel to help reach for the leg.

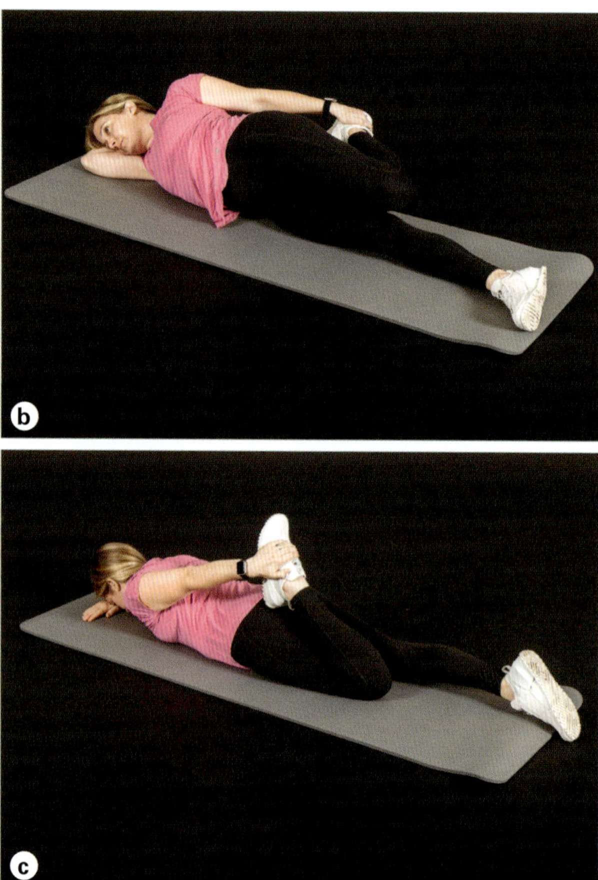

STANDING HAMSTRING STRETCH

Many of my clients experience tight hamstrings. The reason this area may be tight will vary; for some, the body may restrict range of motion here to protect other areas such as the back. Proceed with caution with these stretches and pay attention to how you feel afterward. Adding stability work for the core and back (see stabilizing exercises in chapter 9) may help to release tension overall.

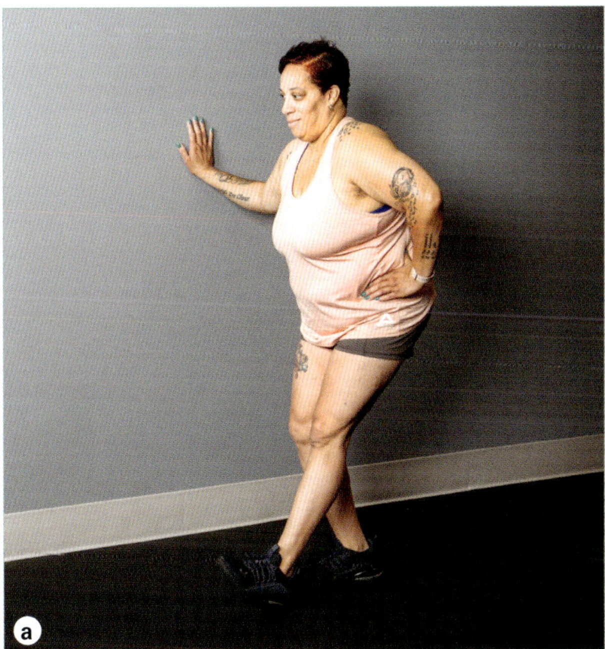

a

Instructions

From a standing position, extend one leg forward and place the heel on the ground. Keep your back straight, shoulders down, and gently hinge forward until you feel a stretch in the straight leg *(a)*. Aim to bring the sit bones up to the ceiling behind you. Place your hands on the supporting leg or on a stable surface. Hold for time, and switch to the other side.

Variations

The hamstrings can also be stretched from a seated position. Sitting at the edge of your chair, extend one leg forward, and lean forward with a straight back until you feel a gentle stretch in the back of the extended leg. Place your hands on the other leg and breathe. This stretch can also be performed lying supine on your back. Bend one knee and straighten the other leg. Hold on to the back of the thigh or calf and gently pull until you feel a gentle stretch *(b)*. Use a strap or towel if it's difficult to hold on to the leg *(c)*.

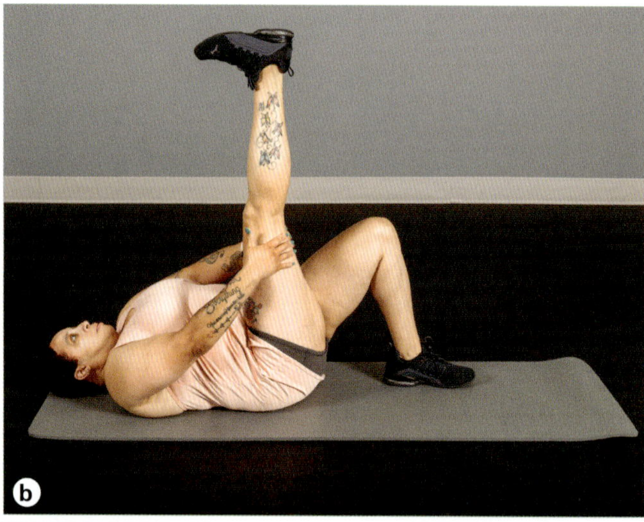
b

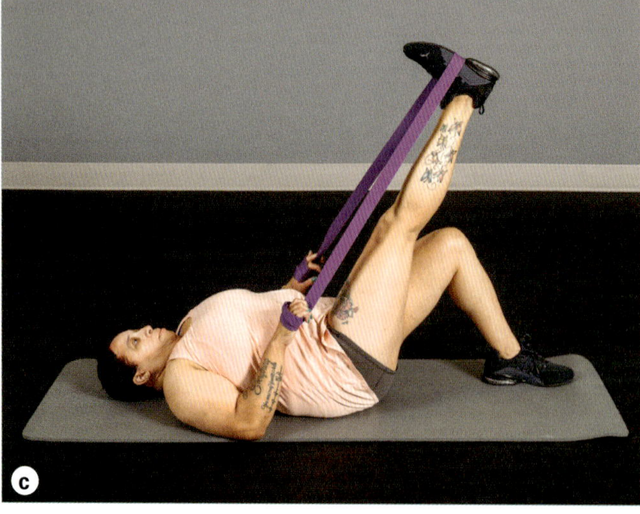
c

STANDING FIGURE 4

This is one of those stretches that either feels very good or the exact opposite. Take your time to move into the stretch and try not to force the range. Use tools to help you feel comfortable and breathe throughout the stretch.

Instructions

From a standing position, hold on to a secure object or wall. Place one ankle above the opposite knee and bend the standing leg. Lean forward with a straight back until you feel a gentle stretch in the hips and glutes of the top leg *(a)*. Hold for time, and switch to the other side.

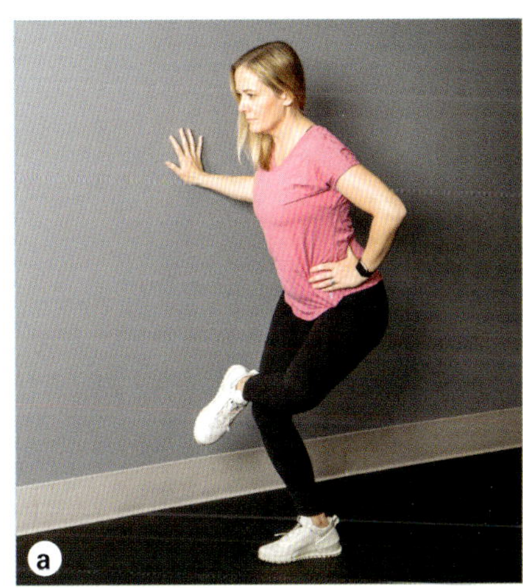

Variations

Try this stretch from a supine position. Lie on your back and bend both knees. Lift both legs and place your left ankle above your right knee. Hold on to your right leg behind the thigh. Pull the legs toward your chest until you feel a gentle hip stretch *(b)*. Move your legs over to the right to feel a deeper stretch toward the outside of the hips *(c)*. Hold for time, and switch to the other side. With the right leg crossed over, shift the legs to the left. If it's difficult to reach for the thigh, place the foot on a chair or ball and keep your arms relaxed by your sides.

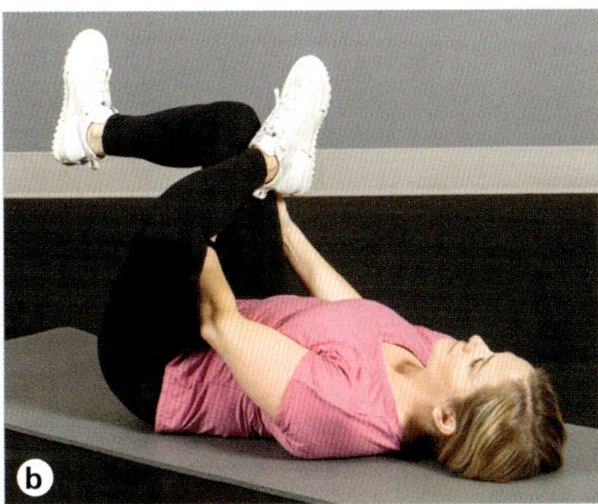

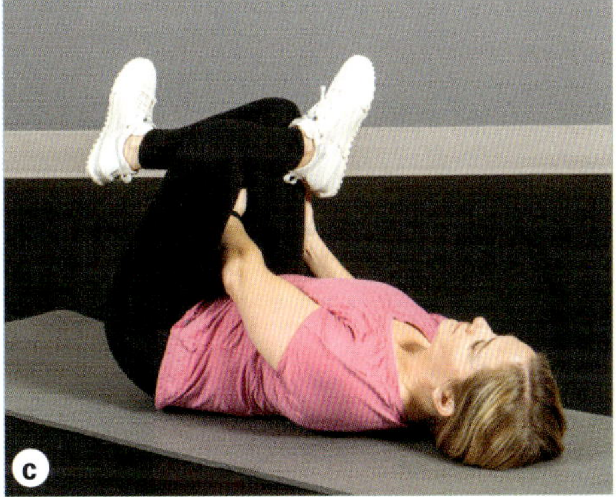

STANDING SHIN STRETCH LUNGE

The shins can feel achy during walking, especially when starting to increase intensity. Try both shin stretches and select the one that feels most effective for you. Ease into both of them and aim to target the midpoint of the shin muscles and not the ankle.

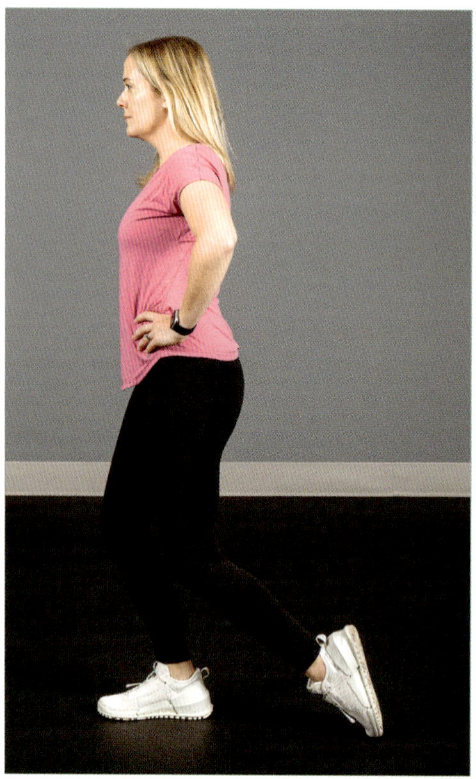

Instructions

From a tall standing position, take a step forward and bend both knees slightly. Flip the foot of the back leg so that your shoelaces face the ground. Think of lengthening the front of the lower leg until you feel a stretch in the back shin or tibialis anterior. Hold for time, then switch to the other side.

Variations

Bend both knees lower to deepen the stretch. Hold on to a wall or stable object for more support.

STANDING SHIN STRETCH CROSS OVER

Ease into this shin stretch, targeting the midpoint of the shin muscles and not the ankle.

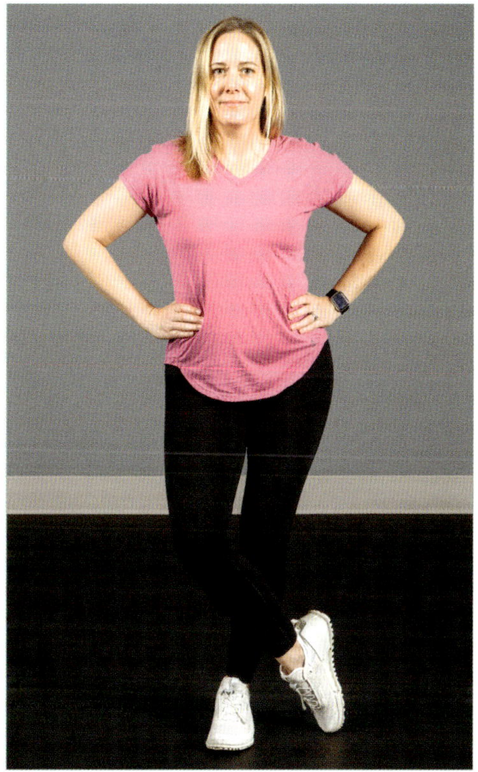

Instructions

From a tall standing position, cross one leg in front of the other and place the foot on the floor. If your right foot is crossed in front, flip your right foot so that your shoelaces or top of your foot is facing down toward the floor. Bend your standing leg and press the shin of that leg into the calf of the front leg to lengthen the front leg. Bend until you feel a gentle stretch in the front shin or tibialis anterior. Hold for time, then switch to the other side.

Variations

Bend both knees lower to deepen the stretch. Hold on to a wall or stable object for more support.

STANDING CHEST STRETCH

Many of us are stuck in a forward, rounded, or internally rotated shoulder position much of the day. Opening the chest and shoulders can create balance in the body and give us an opportunity to stretch tight areas. It's essentially the opposite of how many of us spend our days and can be very effective at improving posture and comfort.

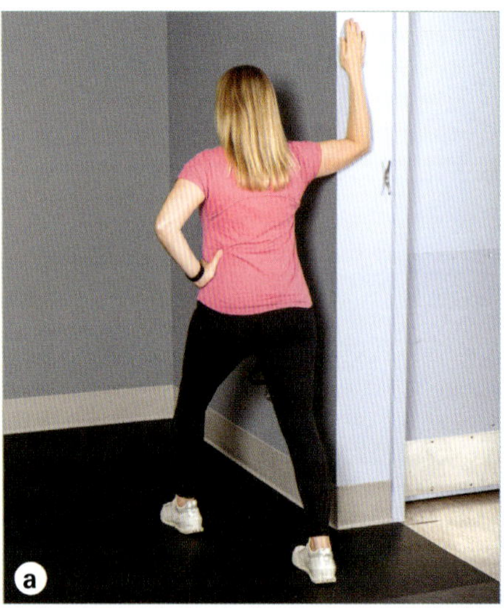

Instructions

Stand tall and place the forearm of one arm along a wall, doorway, or sturdy object. Keep a 90-degree bend in the arm (give or take, depending on comfort) and lean forward slightly until you feel an opening in the chest and shoulders *(a)*. You can place your feet side by side or staggered with one leg back to stretch the calf of the back leg at the same time. Hold for time, then switch to the other side.

Variations

You can stretch both sides at the same time by placing both forearms in a doorway. Stagger your feet and lean forward with a straight back. If you have a doorway at home, you can aim to pause and stretch your chest when walking through *(b)*. This stretch can also be done in a seated position. Sit tall and place your arms gently behind your head. Open your chest, look up slightly, and reach your elbows back until you feel a stretch in your chest *(c)*.

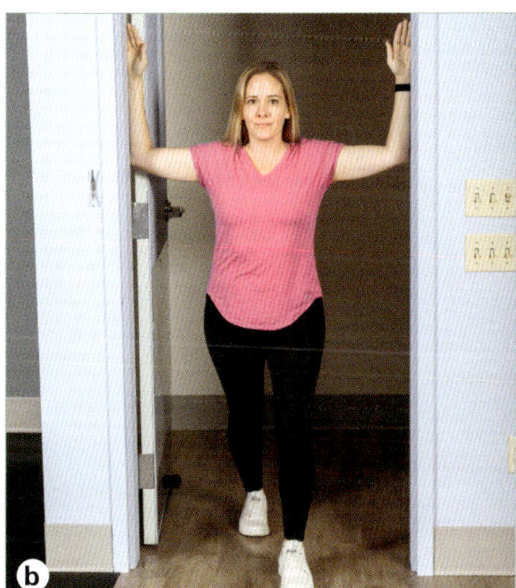
b

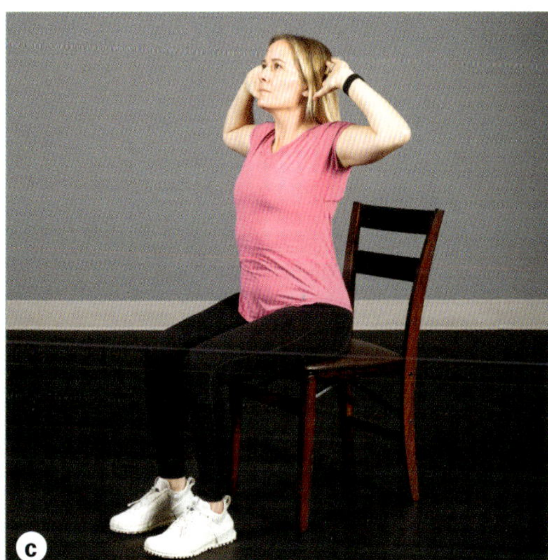
c

BACK STRETCH

For most of us, it would be hard to stretch our backs and feel very little, because most of us have tight zones in some part of our backs, whether low, middle, or high. Explore the different back stretch variations and select the one that feels safest for you. Breathe through the stretch and aim to keep your head and shoulders relaxed.

Instructions

From a standing position, hold on to a post, doorway, or sturdy object with one hand by pronating and placing your hand, thumb down to hold your support. Bend your knees, round your back, and gently pull away to feel a stretch along your back and sides *(a)*. You can lean slightly toward the same-side arm to intensify the stretch. Hold for time, then switch arms.

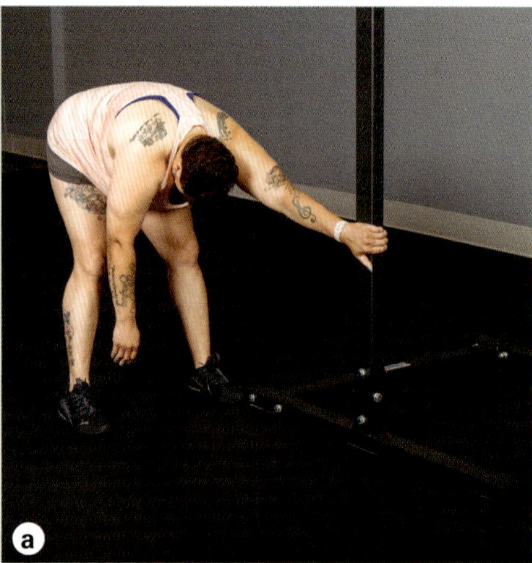
a

Variation

Try this stretch from a seated position if more convenient. Sit at the edge of your chair and bend down to clasp your hands or forearms behind your knees *(b)*. Let your head relax and be heavy.

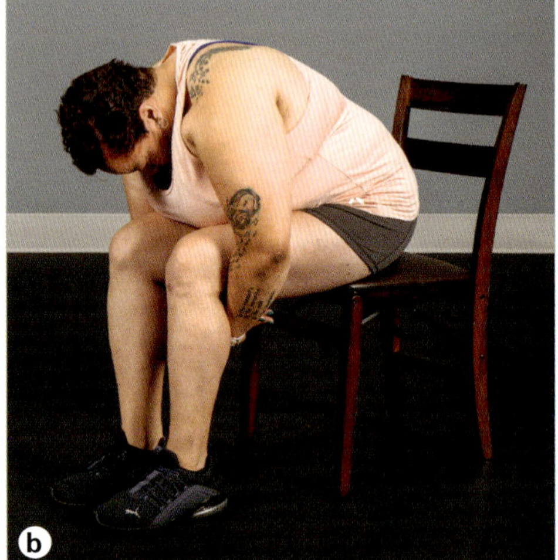
b

STANDING CALF STRETCH

If you are prone to plantar fasciitis, Achilles tendinitis, or chronic tight calves, include this stretch following a walk. Explore the different variations and select the one that targets the area that feels tightest on you. Breathe and stretch this area when your legs are warm. Strengthening this zone builds tissue tolerance, and we'll cover strength exercises for the calves in more detail in chapter 9.

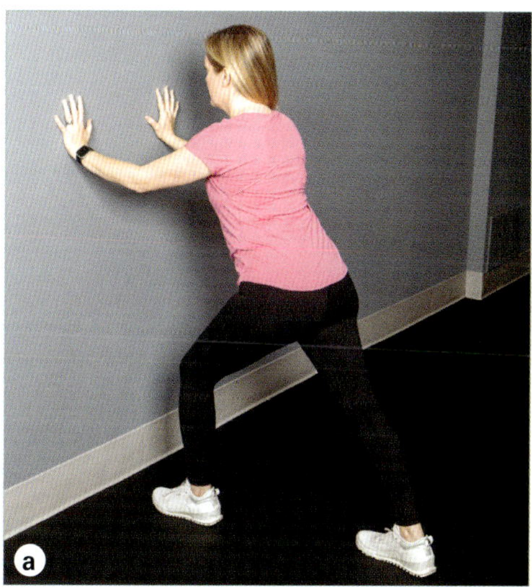

Instructions

Begin by standing tall with your hands on a wall for support. Place one leg back about 3 feet (1 m) and straighten it while bending your front leg. Press your back heel down to the floor until you feel a stretch in the calf area *(a)*. You can bend your back knee slightly to feel the stretch slightly deeper in the soleus muscle. Hold for time, then switch to the other side.

Variations

From the calf stretch position, slowly straighten your front leg and lean forward with a straight back to feel a gentle stretch along both calves *(b)*. You may also feel your hamstring being stretched as well. Alternatively, you can place your feet on a step, step stool, or stable elevated surface and let one heel gently hang off the edge until you feel a stretch on the calf area *(c)*. Ensure you're holding on to something secure for balance.

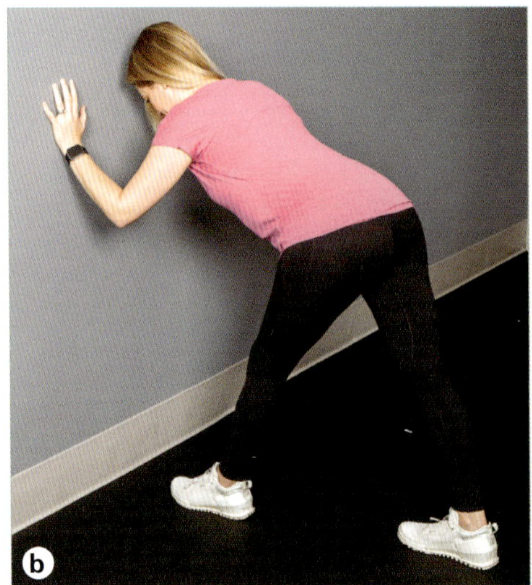

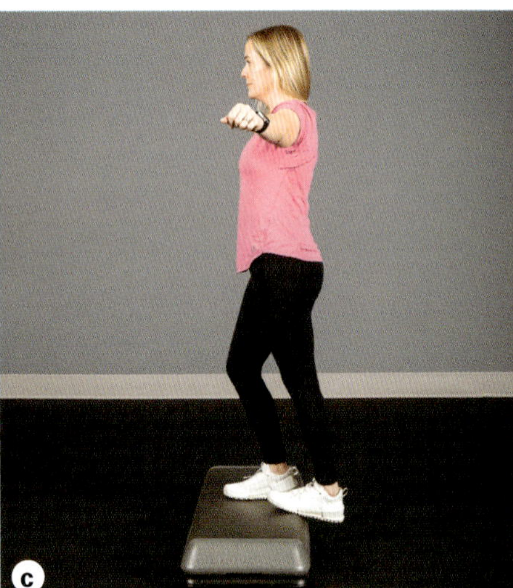

CHILD'S POSE WITH SIDE REACHES

This stretch also targets the back and provides another alternative. Spend some time breathing in this posture, allowing your muscles to relax, after a walk or workout. Use the tools and suggestions to feel comfortable and safe in this stretch. Breathe and enjoy!

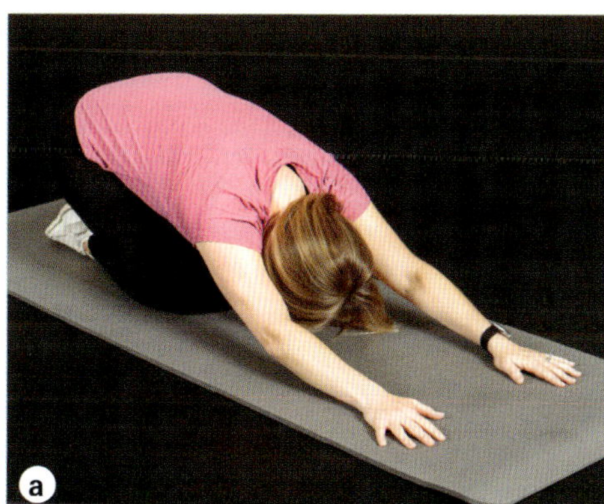
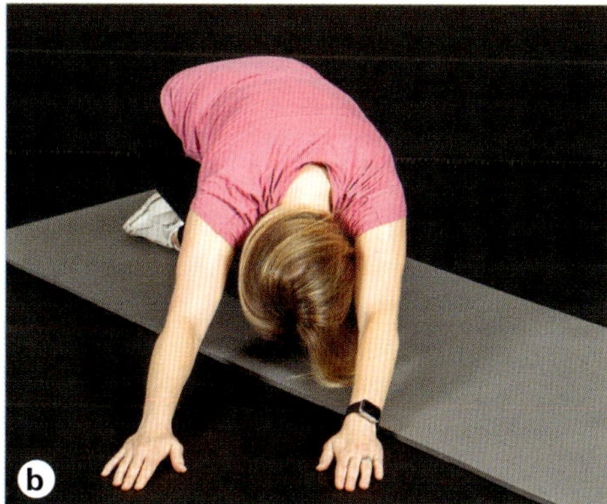

Instructions

Begin in a quadruped all-four's position on a mat with your hands under your shoulders and knees under your hips *(a)*. Untuck your toes and slowly move your hips back toward your heels until you feel a stretch in your back. Relax your head and walk your hands over to one side to feel the stretch along one side *(b)*. Breathe deeply and switch sides.

Variations

Begin as previously instructed but place your head on a support like a pillow or block if it's more comfortable *(c)*. Try placing your knees wider apart to allow for a more comfortable position *(d)*. Your arms can reach forward or rest beside your hips with the palms facing up *(e)*.

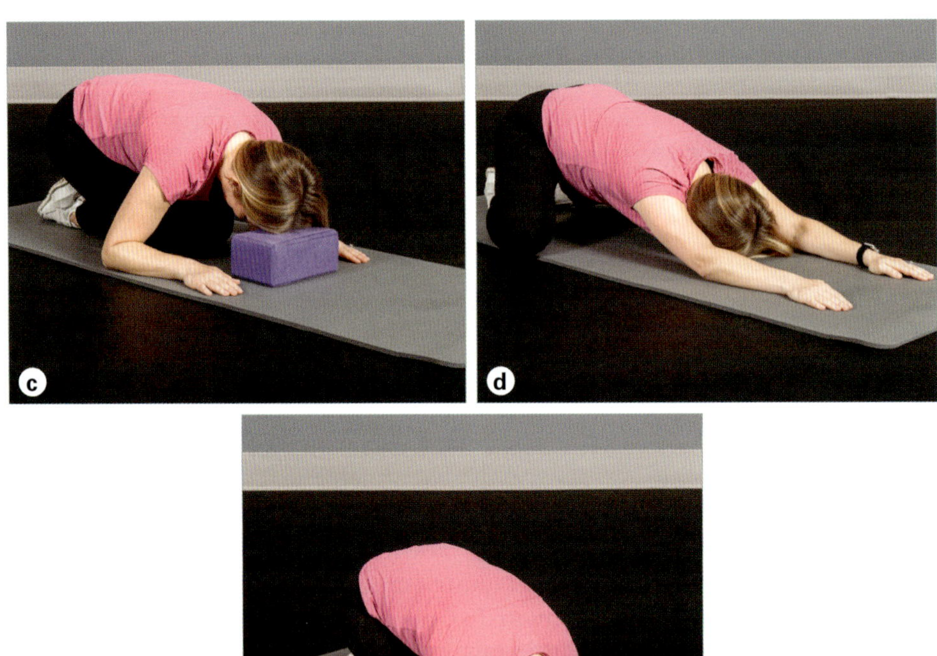

SUPINE PERONEAL STRETCH WITH ROPE OR STRAP

If you tend to supinate or feel tension along the outside edge or lateral line of the lower leg, this stretch can be extra helpful. It works best with shoes on. If you're someone who stretches barefoot or in sock feet, putting shoes on for this stretch may be best. Alternatively, you can perform this stretch first before taking your shoes off for the remainder of your stretch session.

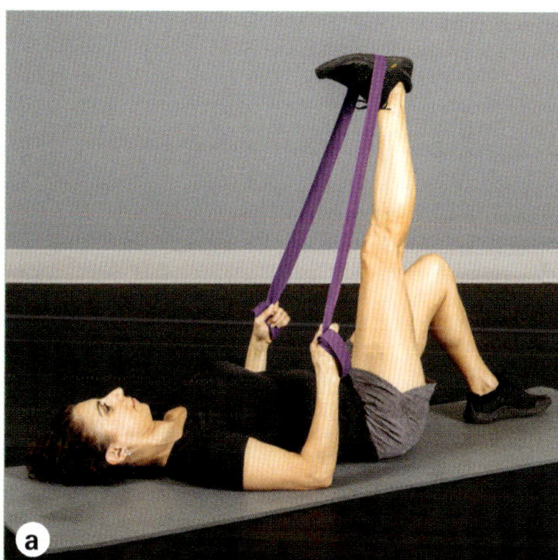
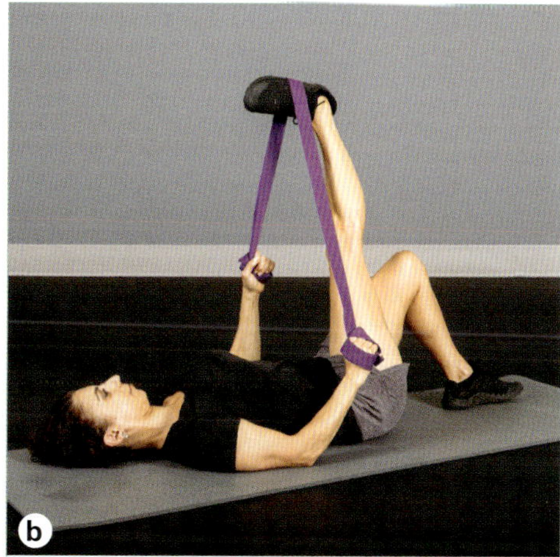

Instructions

Begin by lying on your back with your knees bent. Place a strap, belt, or long towel in the arch of your right foot. Slowly straighten your right leg until you feel a gentle stretch in your hamstrings *(a)*. From there, turn your right foot inward so the sole of the foot now faces the left wall (instead of the ceiling). Gently bring your leg across the body to the left to feel a stretch along the side of the lower leg *(b)*. Hold for time, then switch to the other side.

Variations

Bringing your leg closer to your body and farther across the body will provide a more intense stretch. Gently pull on the inside strap for a deeper peroneal (side of lower leg) stretch.

SUPINE WIPERS WITH TENSOR FASCIAE LATAE (TFL) STRETCH

The outside of the front of the hip can be a tricky area to stretch. I like to combine this gentle spinal twist variation with a stretch for the tensor fascia latae (TFL), the muscle that serves as the insertion point for the IT band. We know that you can stretch your IT band, but not actually lengthen it (Seeber et al. 2020). It may feel best to stretch the insertion of the IT band at the TFL and other surrounding hip muscles.

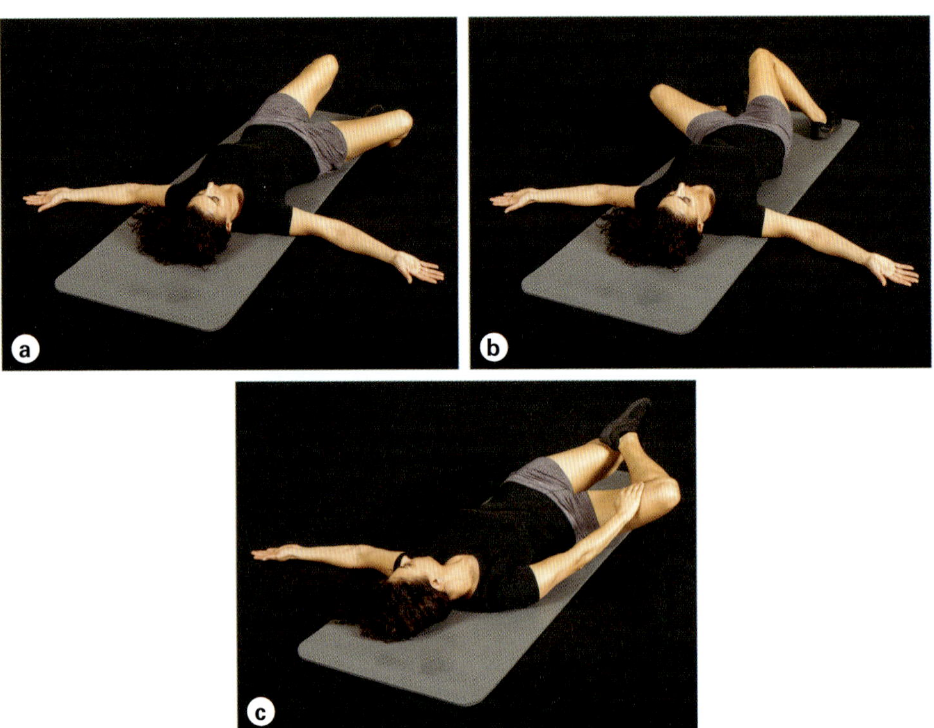

Instructions

Begin by lying on your back with your knees bent and your feet flat on the floor. Your hands can rest by your sides. Gently rock the knees from side to side, pausing in any areas that feel tight or restricted *(a-b)*. You can perform a slow side-to-side motion or move to one side, hold, and repeat on the other side. After the wipers, pause with your knees shifted to one side and pick up your bottom foot. Place the foot on the outside of the top thigh. If your knees are dropped to the right side, pick up your right foot and place it on the left outer thigh *(c)*. Hold for time, then switch to the other side.

Variation

Place your feet wider apart for increased comfort. For a more intense TFL stretch, place your bottom hand on the inner thigh. If your knees are shifted to the left side, place your left hand on your left inner thigh and gently pull the leg down *(d)*. Repeat on the other side.

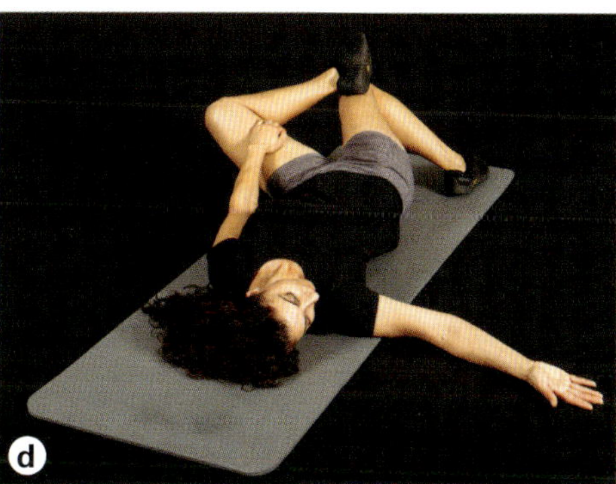

Warming up and cooling down may seem frivolous or time consuming; however, both are important to ensure the brain and body are primed for movement and the heart and blood vessels are recovering from activity. Depending on your injury history, age, daily activity, mobility, and flexibility, it may be necessary to lengthen or shorten the warm-up and cool-down periods and customize them. Using other recovery tools such as foam rollers, therapy balls, massage techniques, and cold or hot therapy can also be effective. Consult with your health care provider for support and advice.

CHAPTER 7

Amplification Tips and Strategies

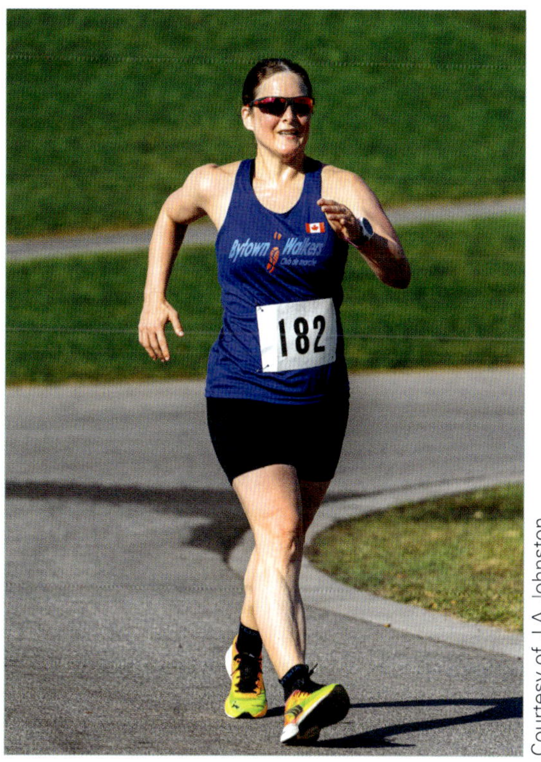

Courtesy of J A Johnston.

Is walking enough? Yes and no. I often speak with people who discount walking as a valid form of cardiovascular activity. They believe it doesn't count. Be assured, with the right strategies and intensity, it counts. From a cardiovascular perspective, when amplified enough and performed to a moderate and vigorous intensity, it counts. Although, if the body allows, working and loading at higher impacts will be beneficial from many standpoints. From a bone density, muscular system, and tissue tolerance perspective, small amounts of jumping and higher-impact activities can help to round out a solid plan. A variety of activities is important to build our threshold and tolerance to all the demands of life. Is walking enough? For some, yes. For others, no. If we're able to elevate our heart rates and ensure we work in a moderate to vigorous zone, yes, it can be enough. Some of my race walking workouts and races elevate my heart rate similar to what running would. But I believe in mixing things up. There's value in walking as well as performing other cardiovascular activities to help build resilience. Personally, I walk, run, sprint, dance, hike, rebound, cycle, and cross-country ski and downhill ski throughout the winter for cardiovascular activity (not typically all in the same week, however).

Balancing out a walking routine with strength training is key for everyone and all bodies. We all need some form of loading to help build and maintain muscle mass, especially as we age. Sarcopenia (muscle loss) is common as we age, especially among women. Maintaining and building muscle mass is critical. Quadriceps strength and grip strength have been correlated with longevity, especially in older populations (Laukkanen et al. 2020; Rijk et al. 2016; Newman et al. 2006; Nakamura et al. 2021).

Before we can work on amplifying and intensifying our walks, it's important to note that walking efficiently will be an important foundation element to perfect before increasing challenge. Walking in an efficient pattern will allow us to walk faster. Landing with our center over our base will be key before adding further challenges.

Speed

It may seem simple: We want to walk faster, so we walk faster. However, the way in which we walk faster will keep our bodies feeling comfortable. Ideally, we want to increase speed by taking short, quick steps. It may seem counterintuitive. We think of the beautiful distance runners who run like gazelles with long strides. "But they have natural talent and often years of training. Watch them carefully and you will see that they are actually landing with their feet directly underneath them. That's what makes their strides efficient. They are long, but not too long," says Roger Burrows, race walking coach and founder of the Bytown Walkers. As we increase speed, keeping our center of gravity over our center of mass will help us to modulate and absorb ground forces more effectively. In other words, landing with our foot underneath us will keep us stable and allow us to use our muscles more efficiently.

Overstriding is one of the most common errors I see in walking form, especially in people who experience low back pain. Taking a larger step puts more strain on our low backs and can slow us down. When we take too big of a stride, we land with our foot essentially in front of us, not under us. The back, legs, and hips take the brunt of the load. Try it: Walk around with overexaggerated large strides and pay attention to how your back feels. Then, take smaller steps and reassess. The smaller strides allow us to walk more efficiently, landing with our center over our base and giving our core muscles the chance to support us well. Burrows shares, “From a standing position, move your foot as if you were pushing on the brake pedal in a car. You can actually feel the braking action through the leg and into the body. We don’t want to have to haul ourselves over a leg stretched forward. We want the feet to be moving backward when we contact the ground.” Smaller strides will also help us move into a speedy rhythm. Quick steps and a fast turnover give us opportunities to push away from the ground more frequently. Our first step in increasing walking speed is taking quicker, faster, shorter steps.

Another strategy to increase walking speed is to use the arms. We learned in the gait chapter to hold our arms in a comfortably bent position—similar to running arms. While maintaining this fixed position, drive the elbows back with a little more emphasis. The backward arm drive will help to create forward momentum. Similar to a slingshot, the focus is on creating backward recoil to propel an object forward. We don’t want to punch the arms forward in front of us to help us walk faster. It’s the backward elbow drive that gives us that added push. When holding the arms in the bent position—aim to keep the palms facing inward and the forearms moving back and forth generally parallel to the ground. This ensures the shoulders remain in a fairly neutral position and in a less internally rotated forward setup. This allows us to use our posterior shoulder, rotator cuff, and back a bit more effectively.

We can also think of pushing down into the ground with the feet with a slightly stronger emphasis. After the foot hits the ground and moves closer to being directly underneath us, think of pushing the foot down into the ground. This will help to prime the hip extension pattern, create more awareness around the hip extensors such as the glutes and hamstrings, and propel us forward faster. Every action has an equal and opposite reaction. “When we push against the ground, the ground pushes back, therefore moving us forward. Essentially the only time we move ourselves forward is as a result of our contact with the ground,” shares Burrows. The downward push does not have to be aggressively strong. A light push off will work well so as not to lose forward momentum but help with a stronger, quicker drive.

Practice some of these elements outdoors or indoors on stable surfaces, then explore using a treadmill (if accessible) to help increase walking speed. Although walking mechanics are different on a treadmill versus stable surfaces, it can be a tool to help our bodies feel what it’s like to walk faster. After warming up on a treadmill, aim to slowly increase walking speed. Pause at a comfortable pace that feels similar to your outdoor walking pace. Once you’ve held that for a few minutes, try walking a little faster. What do you notice? What has to happen to help your body walk faster? Make note of the arms, legs, feet, and overall pace and rhythm.

Incorporating those changes and elements into your next outdoor walk may help you to explore a faster walking pace.

Although we are referring to speed in a more general sense of walking at a quick pace, we really should refer to it in more specific terms. When increasing our walking pace, many elements must fall into place to allow us to maintain our alignment, position, mechanics, muscle contractions, and positioning with good form and ease. Our speed may not be simply walking as fast as we can but rather "as quick as we know we can comfortably maintain for the duration of our walk. In walking terms, that concept is important enough to have its own specific word: rhythm," explains Burrows.

Walking faster essentially entails having the ability to have good strength and stamina to maintain our desired walking rhythm over time. With good cardiovascular and muscular endurance and strength, we're able to maintain our desired walking rhythm for longer periods. Walking faster means the heart and muscles have good strength and endurance. That foundation of strength and endurance will over time help us increase our walking speed for a short distance—and, more important, our rhythm for as long as we decide to walk!

Hills

One of my favorite ways to amplify any walk is to add some form of elevation. Whether it's a hill within a neighborhood, a hilly hike in the forest, or a stairwell, adding some form of hill training will help to intensify your walk and surely make it count. Hill training will help to increase strength and later on, speed or rhythm. Studies have shown that walking on a 5 to 10 percent incline uses more muscle recruitment than walking on a level surface and strengthens the knee joint (Haggerty et al. 2014).

To start, select a small hill within your neighborhood. You may have limited access to hills, but if you live in or frequent an area with some hills, explore this option. Walk up the hill at a slower pace than your regular walking pace. Once you reach the top, walk down to the bottom slowly. Take a short walking break if needed, and repeat the hill climb again. Over time, work on walking faster up the hill. When that feels comfortable, explore walking up longer or steeper hills. Add one variable at a time (e.g., steepness, speed, height of hill) and progress slowly from there.

Walking downhill will put more strain on the quadriceps and knees. If you experience some discomfort in the knees when descending, try dynamic stretches beforehand (the walking hip flexor dynamic stretch and a short static stretch for the quadriceps group found in chapter 6 would work well). Try adding a gentle core contraction when stepping down in an effort to offload the knees. Slowing down the walking pace, planting with the heel first, using walking poles on the descent, or walking sideways if comfortable can be safer alternatives to explore.

If you don't have access to hills, a stairwell, aerobic step, or plyometric box are options. Walk up the stairs slowly, being mindful of planting the full foot on the stair to minimize calf strain. Push through the heel as you step up to engage the posterior chain such as the glutes and hamstrings. Start with one flight of steps and aim to add additional flights or repeat the flight over time. Walk down slowly to recover in between sets. If going downstairs is bothersome on your knees, use an elevator if available to go down or step down sideways while you build up knee tolerance.

If you have an aerobic step or similar secure platform, repeating a stepping pattern can also work to increase intensity. Plant the full foot on your step and aim to push through the midfoot and heel to come up. Step down lightly and repeat with the other leg. Your stepping pattern can mimic climbing a hill by alternating legs, similar to a walking pattern. The variation is shown in figure 7.1. If repeating the same side is most comfortable, that can also be a great option.

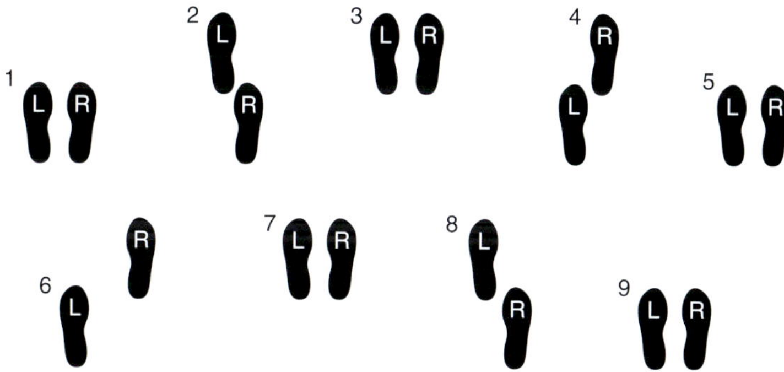

FIGURE 7.1 Diagram of stepping pattern on step, stair, or secure object.

Some form of incline work can help to increase overall effort, cardiovascular output, and muscular challenge. Hills, treadmills, stairs, aerobic steps, or plyometric boxes provide options to perform some form of hill training. The overall results are numerous; the ease of climbing your next flight of stairs may surprise you with consistent hill training.

Intervals

Interval training is an excellent variable used to amplify intensity. Interval training comes in many forms: Fartlek, high-intensity interval training (HIIT), spring interval training (SIT), Tabata, and every minute on the minute (EMOM), or as many reps as possible (AMRAP) are some of the more popular forms.

In general, high-intensity interval training has been shown to improve $\dot{V}O_2max$, resting metabolic rate, body composition, insulin sensitivity, and cognitive functions. Our $\dot{V}O_2max$ is a measurement of cardiovascular fitness and aerobic endurance. High-intensity exercise has also been shown to decrease the risk for cardiovascular disease, breast cancer, metabolic syndrome, osteoarthritis, and rheumatoid arthritis known to cause low back pain (Atakan et al. 2021). Interval walking training can increase physical fitness in middle-aged and older people (Masuki et al. 2017). Interval training has been proven more effective than moderate-intensity training on glucose control (Mendes et al. 2019). Selecting intervals over moderate-intensity exercise yields greater cardiorespiratory fitness results. We essentially receive a bigger bang for our buck with shorter, more-intense bouts of exercise, walking included.

With walking, we can keep interval training simple. After a thorough warm-up, increase walking speed for 20 to 60 seconds, followed by walking at a slower pace to recover for 90 seconds to 2 minutes (or longer if needed). Repeat this format 5 to 10 times and finish with a cool-down and stretch. The interval portion of the walk should be challenging and difficult. The goal is to elevate the heart rate, increase the overall demand, and challenge our systems so that we fatigue at the end of our 20-, 30-, or 60-second interval. Ideally, we need the full recovery walk to gear up for the next interval.

If looking at your watch or device is challenging or disruptive, select a landmark ahead on your path and aim to increase walking speed or rhythm until you reach that specific object (e.g., light post, tree, building). The timing doesn't have to be specific when starting out. We'll include more detailed interval walking plans in chapter 11. The idea is to remain consistent, ensure there are distinctions between the interval and recovery period, and work to progressively increase intensity and/or number of intervals over time.

Varying Terrain

Changing our stimulus in day-to-day movements is beneficial in providing new challenges to our bones, joints, muscles, tendons, sensory nerves, and tissues. Walking on a beach barefoot provides a different challenge than walking on asphalt in supportive footwear. Mixing things up and providing different challenges trains our systems to handle various terrains with more ease. It may take some time to work up to walking in different terrains; however, with consistent practice, our feet and bodies will adapt.

We can explore changing the terrain where possible within our overall training week. More of your walks can be performed on stable outdoor surfaces such as asphalt and cement. If you consistently walk indoors, treadmills or large indoor walking areas can make up the bulk of your mileage. When possible, walk on slightly different surfaces and see how things feel. It could be a walking trail, a gravel or dirt road, a sandy beach, a grassy area, a snowy trail, or rocky terrain. Adjust footwear and clothing depending on personal needs, temperature, and terrain.

The more we challenge norms and routines, the more capable we are of handling our contact surface. Our brains remember "we've been here before," and feel a sense of stability and comfort with prior exposures. The results of varying walking surfaces will yield a more dynamic, versatile, adaptable, and stable system.

Load

Rucking is currently a trend that is gaining a lot of attention. Rucking is essentially walking with a weighted vest (or pack) to add an additional challenge to our walks or hikes. Maybe you've had opportunities to carry heavier loads and realize that the effort required is much greater. Examples include going to the grocery store for one thing and leaving with two heavy bags to carry home or lugging a sleeping baby in a carrier while walking or, even more challenging, a squirming toddler! Perhaps you've been on a hike while carrying a backpack. These are examples of opportunities where carrying additional load provides a greater challenge output while walking. We feel the additional effort as we may be breathing heavier, sweating more, or finding the movement feels more intense. Studies have shown that walking with 10 percent of your body weight in a backpack on your back will increase your overall rate of perceived exertion (Sen and Singh 2016).

Opportunities in our day-to-day lives add more challenge while adding additional load, such as carrying children, hiking with extra weight, performing farmer's carries (carrying load in one or each hand) in the gym or at home, or walking home with extra bags to increase the challenge. Or we can purposefully increase our load while walking to amplify our workout. We don't have many studies with healthy populations (with strong methodologies and large group sizes) to fully support the use of weighted walking at the time of publication, yet there may be value in sometimes adding load to our walks to build a robust system to tolerate daily demands that may require you to walk with heavier loads.

Start by carrying a well-fitted backpack or weighted vest, focusing on increasing the load slowly and progressively. Ideally, start very light, such as a couple of pounds to begin. From there, work to increase the load slowly on a weekly basis if consistent and comfortable. For the average walker, add a maximum of 10 percent of our body weight. Even with adding 10 percent of our body weight in a vest or pack, we will see changes in gait mechanics and added hip movements and activations, such as greater hip flexion (Wang et al. 2023).

Walking with weights in your hands or walking with ankle weights is not recommended. When using weights, we ideally want to move through slow, controlled movements while avoiding momentum for a certain number of repetitions. We can perform a biceps curl in a slow controlled manner, for example, for 8 to 12 repetitions, and rest and repeat for a few sets. The added repeated load in the extremities when weighted while walking can cause discomfort in the shoulders and other joints that may not be able to support the load over time. Our gait mechanics can be altered, and this may lead to injury. Walk with the load closer to your body versus in your hands or on your ankles for joint comfort and safety.

Walking with load may not be for everyone. For those who can tolerate added loads, it may help build a resilient system where over time, carrying objects while walking becomes easier. Aim to increase either load or distance at one time. Try to focus on increasing one variable at a time, such as speed, load, intensity, or terrain, to avoid injury or discomfort.

Many may discount walking as a legitimate form of exercise, but it certainly counts, especially with the amplification tips and strategies outlined in this chapter. Aim to incorporate these challenges, one element at a time, and see how your body feels. In the next chapter, we'll discuss modifications and injury prevention tips.

CHAPTER 8

Modifications and Injury Prevention

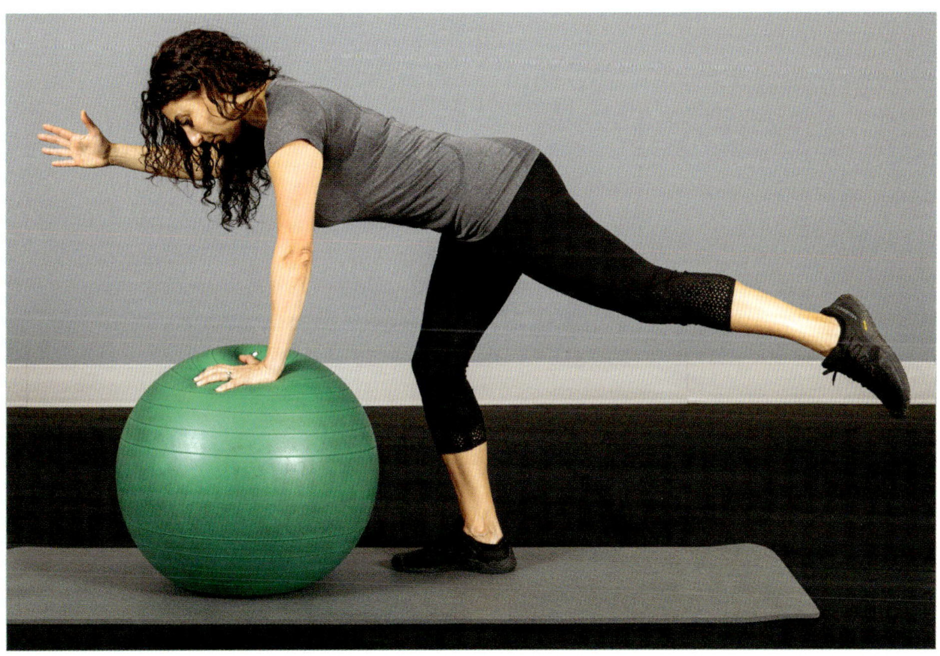

It happens. We get injured, sidetracked, off course, and life can get in the way of our consistent routine. Walking consistently is what will help us reap all the benefits outlined in chapter 1. Walking occasionally won't get us there. When we're injured, it's difficult to remain consistent. There are, however, solutions to help us stay on track when we're not at our best or are out of our normal routine. There's always something we can do. It might entail reducing our volume, intensity, time, or adjusting footwear. It may require us to adjust our form and technique. It may require more purposeful warm-up, cool-down, and preparatory and corrective movements to help us move forward. It can all be done to bridge the gap back to our normal.

Modifications

Sometimes it is necessary to modify our workouts, plan ahead, or pivot in order to remain consistent in our efforts. Consistency will be the first element helping us to see results and automate our walking routines. Adjusting our sessions when the weather is less than ideal or when traveling will help us remain on track. Modify as necessary to stay in the game. You might need to include less volume or intensity, train at a different time, use a different modality (e.g., treadmill), adjust plans, add in recovery strategies, or change your gear slightly to adjust to weather or travel situations that interrupt usual routines. If we can make things work in any situation, routines become more automated and eventually require less effort, bandwidth, or thought. We just go, no matter what.

Weather

Living in Canada means winters are unpredictable. Snow, ice, cold, and wind are common issues for Canadians during winter months. Other countries and cities may be similar. If we always waited for the perfect weather day to walk, it would be difficult to remain consistent. Despite the weather, we can arm ourselves with the right tools and dress for success. We discussed clothing and the importance of fabrics, layers, quality, and protection in more detail in chapter 3.

I may skip outdoor walking when it's –30 degrees Celsius, but I'll aim to dress warmly and head out when it's not as bitter. I may opt for an indoor format if conditions are very icy. It's important to be adaptable, versatile, open, and flexible because the weather is largely out of our control. What variables can we control? To an extent, clothing, timing (waiting until it warms up later in the day or walking earlier in the morning if too hot), and location are variables we can alter to ensure we remain consistent. Look for the windows of opportunity to present themselves and take advantage. Can you walk while your kids participate in organized sports? Can you walk and talk with your coworker outside instead of sitting in a meeting room? Can you listen to a podcast while walking?

Overall, it's okay to skip those unfavorable weather days if it's unsafe and uncomfortable. Aim for consistency, and try to get back on track. The extreme cold and hot weather days may be a perfect opportunity to focus on strength training (chapter 9).

Travel

For many of us, travel is enjoyable and relaxing and often includes plenty of walking (through airports, touring new sights, getting to your destination). Walking tours are offered in many countries as a way to explore and learn. Although we may be out of our regular walking and exercise routines, research and ask about routes and walkable pathways at your destination. Where are safe areas that you can explore on foot? Are trails, walking paths, and clear sidewalks within close distance to your hotel or place of stay? Speaking with the local population, spending some time online in advance, and asking the hotel concierge or homeowner about possible routes and locations will help you plan out an active and walkable trip.

Many hotels have gyms and wellness centers (or easy access to fitness centers) as part of their community networking initiatives. Using the treadmill in the hotel fitness center is a great way to keep to your walking routine while traveling. If your hotel doesn't have an on-site fitness center or access to one, walking around the hotel can also be an option as well as using the stairs for a quick, intense bouts of physical activity. Aiming to fit in small exercise snacks can help to keep your walking fitness up while you're traveling.

Common Walking Injuries

You may experience initial discomforts when beginning a new exercise plan. Walking should not be painful. You may experience stiffness or soreness in the form of delayed onset of muscle soreness (DOMS) in the day or two following a new, different, or more intense activity. The muscle soreness is not a direct indication of how hard you worked, and we shouldn't use it as a barometer of how well your workout went. You may find yourself feeling a bit more uncomfortable after certain walks, especially on new terrain, at higher volumes, on closer walking intervals, and at faster speeds.

The following examples are some of the more common walking injuries we will hopefully *not* encounter. The majority are overuse injuries, although overuse can be different based on the individual. Overuse is essentially the body's inability to withstand the demands placed upon it, and we need to increase thresholds and ceilings so our bodies can withstand the new demands. The general overview here is brief, so please consult your health care practitioner for specific guidance and treatment.

Shin Splints

Shin splints are characterized by pain and inflammation along the medial or lateral aspect of the lower leg, typically caused by overuse and repetitive stress on the tibia (lower leg bone) as well as the connective tissues that attach to the tibia. Because of the repetitive nature and impact of walking, walkers may be prone to shin splints. With overuse, we may feel pain and discomfort. Dr. Taryn Taylor, sports medicine physician and co-owner and medical director of the Carleton Sports Medicine Clinic in Ottawa, Canada, shares, "Shin splints are on the MTSS (medial tibial stress syndrome) spectrum and should be managed appropriately to ensure it doesn't progress to a stress fracture. Treatments include modified activities, cross-training, water-based activities, and physiotherapy. Compression stockings or shin splint sleeves can also offer some relief and allow walking to continue."

Work to avoid shin splints by gradually progressing walking volume; walking with proper footwear; adjusting and varying walking surfaces where possible, including a robust warm-up and cool-down; using recovery strategies; building strength and endurance in the lower leg; and seeking treatment and guidance at the first sign of pain or discomfort.

Hip Pain

I remember feeling a small amount of hip discomfort when I first started race walking. This quickly went away as I adapted to the new form of walking. We may experience tight hip muscles with increased distances, intensities, and frequencies. Some may experience greater trochanteric pain syndrome (GTPS), which is characterized by pain in the lateral hip area. Strong gluteal muscles are important to support the hip joint. A strong core and well-coordinated pelvic floor muscles are important to maintain optimal pelvic positioning. If you're feeling tight, an extended warm-up, some dynamic activation of the important hip and core muscles, and a good cool-down and stretching routine focused on the muscles of the hip may help. If the hip pain does not go away, worsens, or changes, see a professional to rule out other hip injuries.

Knee Pain

Some individuals may experience knee pain when walking. Patellofemoral syndrome, a condition that involves pain at the front of the knee, is common in walkers and runners, especially in females due to anatomical differences from males, hormonal factors, knee laxity, and neuromuscular factors (Vora et al. 2018). Iliotibial band syndrome is another common condition affecting the knees, specifically pain on the outside of the knee. We may see more instances of iliotibial band syndrome with hill work. According to Dr. Taylor, "It's important to focus on proper knee mechanics and address muscle imbalances to help with overall knee function." Strengthening areas such as the quadriceps, vastus medialis oblique (VMO), gluteus medius, core musculature, and foot stabilizers will help with overall knee function and pain. We cover exercises to help strengthen these areas in chapter 9.

Back Pain

Eighty percent of people will experience back pain at some point in their lives; that's four of every five people. Although common, it can be debilitating, frustrating, and disheartening. Back pain is a tricky one. The primary driver behind back pain varies and may be due to multiple factors. A weak core, tight hip flexors, poor pelvic positioning, poor alignment, compensatory patterns, weak back muscles, improper firing and timing of muscles, improper lifting or bending mechanics, mismanagement of intra-abdominal pressures, disc issues, surgery, or compression issues may all contribute to causes of low back pain, although pinpointing an exact cause is difficult. There may be additional factors such as stress levels, smoking, metabolic health, socioeconomic factors, system inflammatory conditions such as endometriosis, and current pain beliefs. Addressing symptoms, improving breathing mechanics, optimizing alignment and positioning during movement, increasing strength (core, back, and overall), and loading progressively may all help to restore healthy back function. For many, untreated back pain doesn't always go away quickly. Seek help and guidance if you're experiencing chronic back pain.

Foot Pain

Foot pain may be one of the more common complaints when ramping up walking volume, intensity, and duration. Our feet are incredible structures and withstand a tremendous amount of load throughout the day. Feet may feel sore, tight, uncomfortable, or throbby after a long day on our feet. "Metatarsalgia, Morton's neuromas, or metatarsal stress fractures would be common sources of foot pain in walkers," shares Dr. Taylor. Wearing proper footwear, stretching and rolling out the bottoms of our feet, resting and elevating as a recovery strategy, and using ice or heat if it brings comfort may all be in your foot care toolkit.

Plantar Fasciitis

The word itself can bring a sense of dread to those who have experienced plantar fasciitis firsthand. The plantar fascia attaches to the heel bone. With repetitive heel striking and overuse, this area can become inflamed and painful. We may feel pain when first walking (in the morning or when we first head out the door for our walk). As with most soft tissue overuse injuries, things are uncomfortable at the beginning and may go away or lessen when the tissues are warmed up. This does not mean we should ignore the pain. Proper assessment and treatment are encouraged. Rest and ice have been used traditionally but we now know that tissue responds well to loading. Dr. Taylor says, "The approach to tendon management is to stimulate healing. Where tendons insert into bone is a flaw in our design as there is inadequate blood flow. As a result, current management strategies have moved away from anti-inflammatories and instead toward reactivating the healing cascade." Appropriate loading, mobilization, modified rest, and other strategies will ensure tissue is remodeled and on its way to healing. It does, however, take time. This injury requires quick intervention, serious dedication and consistency with strengthening and stretching, ensuring we're not overloading the area, and using recovery strategies wisely.

Achilles Tendinopathies

Another tricky and frustrating overuse injury, Achilles tendinitis is essentially an inflamed Achilles tendon. The repetitive nature of walking movements, the reliance on the calf, shin, and foot muscles, and the possible ease of overtraining can play a role in this injury. "Similar to plantar fasciitis, management options shift once it becomes chronic (>6 weeks)," according to Dr. Taylor. "After 4 to 6 weeks the inflammatory stage halts and we move into the chronic phase when the tendon is thickened and disorganized and stops trying to heal on its own. This is when treatment options expand into options that stimulate healing such as dry needling, shock wave therapy, nitro patches, or even PRP [platelet-rich plasma therapy]." Strengthening the surrounding muscles and building tissue tolerance will be valuable and helpful. Concentric, eccentric, and isometric calf raises with the appropriate load can be an effective strategy to help build tolerance of the tissues. Be sure you're properly diagnosed, taking your rehabilitation seriously, and stretching and strengthening consistently to improve the tissue threshold required for higher volumes and impacts.

Speak with your health care provider to find your customized solutions to help bridge the gap from injury to a return to pain-free movement.

Return From Injury

Recovering from an injury can be a frustrating experience. Resting or modifying activities when you're someone who is usually active and busy can be a difficult endeavor. We are creatures of habit, and our routines are important to us. We check off that mental box, get a hit of dopamine, and feel good about what we've accomplished. We can almost always recover from musculoskeletal injuries; although the process may vary, overall, we can be strategic with our recovery. The following suggestions can help to speed up your recovery process and ease any anxiety in not being able to perform at 100 percent.

- **Consult with a professional.** When you are injured or suspect an injury, see a professional as soon as possible. Guessing what is wrong or performing a Google search may not be in your best interest. Obtain a proper and professional diagnosis so that you can recover faster. I've often heard from clients who waited, assuming the pain would just go away and heal on its own. Sometimes this is absolutely the case. However, if pain or function is not improving after a few days, it warrants a visit to the doctor or registered physiotherapist (or other qualified diagnostician). From there, they usually prescribe a short period of rest, which may include a day or a few days. Long periods of rest are usually discouraged (unless the injury is severe), because returning to some form of movement is ideal to begin the healing process.
- **Do your rehab.** After receiving a diagnosis, you may be prescribed a series of strength or stability exercises, stretches, or mobility drills with specific repetitions, intervals, rest periods, and intensity levels. Being consistent and prioritizing your rehabilitative exercise will ensure a return to your normal activity levels faster. For some, performing these corrective exercises prior to a walk or activity may help the movement feel more comfortable. Adjust the timing and find what works best, but be consistent to ensure healing and recuperation.
- **Stay active.** When injured, there is always something that can be done. If we can't walk, maybe we can bike. If we can't bike, maybe we can swim. If we can't swim, maybe we can stretch. If we can't lift our usually heavy weights, maybe we can lift lighter or work other body parts while we recover. There is always something. It may take some creativity and consulting with the pros, but find out what you can do, even if it's different or not your preferred activity. Doing something can get the blood moving, makes our bodies feel good, and hastens recovery.
- **Walk if and how you can.** While you are cross-training and healing, you may be able to continue to walk at shorter intervals. When you are walking, progress slowly and gradually to your usual walking pace, distance, and intensity. Start with a baseline that you know is doable. It may be short, but you need a starting point. It might be 5 minutes (or shorter) and that's okay! With a baseline established, increase the distance or time by 10 percent each week. It will feel slow, but it will allow the tissues to acclimate and build and subsequently create new baselines.
- **Focus on form.** Paying close attention to walking form can play a role in preventing injuries over time. When returning from an injury or if you're currently injured, focusing on your walking form and technique can help mitigate the potential discomforts you may be feeling. Proper posture, gait mechanics, technique, and stride length will all help you to feel comfortable and allow you to keep walking. You may have to take smaller steps, walk at slower speeds, or walk for less time, but the

smaller, less intense walking bouts will help you to stay on track overall and maintain your walking regime.

- **Consider alternative footwear.** In the instances of foot and ankle injuries, altering footwear may be required in the short term to give us additional support. That extra bit of cushioning and reinforcement may allow us to walk for longer distances without pain or discomfort. An insole, orthotic, or more supportive shoe may help to offload some of the foot and ankle stabilizers short term, allowing you to remain active. If I experience the beginnings of plantar fasciitis or Achilles tendinitis or if my feet are feeling achy, I'll sometimes opt for a more robust shoe with added support (and a higher heel to forefoot drop). It buys me a bit of extra time to recover, heal, and offload while I remain active on my feet. This is typically done in conjunction with mobilizing and strengthening work and seeking treatment.
- **Use poles for walking assistance.** Walking poles may help to offload some weight and allow us to continue walking. Hiking poles, Nordic walking poles, or other types of poles may provide additional support, decrease pressure on joints, improve overall stability and balance, and help with posture and alignment. Malin Svensson, founder of Nordic Body and author of *Nordic Walking*, shares this:

> Adding two poles using the correct Nordic walking technique while walking is like having two extra legs. Instead of distributing all your weight onto your legs, you now can take stress off your ankles, knees, hips, and lower back with the poles. Especially when you walk down a hill. Bend your knees (mini-squat position), take shorter steps, and lean back onto the poles. Yes, your arms will definitely work harder. Getting used to walking with two poles (Nordic walking) has so many more benefits in your recovering phase as well as after your rehab. You'll feel more stable and thus more confident. Your posture improves the second you apply pressure down (action) through the poles to Mother Earth. The energy (reaction) will travel up the spine, pulling the invisible string from the crown of your head up toward the sky. It's a built-in posture phenomenon with Nordic walking. Last but not least, being outdoors and connecting with nature has a healing effect on your mental and emotional health. Being injured is stressful. Take the time to Nordic walk and you'll feel, after a while, the meditative and calming effect kick in to de-stress your whole body inside and out. Nordic walking generates a specific rhythm (feet and poles hitting the ground) and when you get into the zone you'll feel the meditative effect from that rhythm. In addition, it's very grounding. Every time the poles hit the ground you connect with Mother Earth and feel grounded right away.

• **Emphasize warm-ups and cool-downs.** Take the time to warm up well and stretch afterward. If you're symptomatic when increasing volume, move back to your baseline and increase from there. It can be a frustrating process, but in my 25-plus years of experience, I have found that those who are consistent and who progress slowly are those who are the most successful. There is nothing more frustrating than doing too much too soon and being back at square one.

Once you've built up to your full activities again, think of maintaining as best as possible. Incorporating longer warm-ups and cool-downs in the short term might be helpful. Focus on strength, stability, and mobility to address any underlying weaknesses, compensatory patterns, or issues. Be mindful of what you're feeling, and stop and rest for short periods if needed. Include some reflection. What caused the initial injury? Did you ignore the warning signs? Did you do too much? Can you train smarter to prevent a future recurrence? What can you do now to build a more robust system? Strength, smart progressions, listening to your body, and resting when in doubt are the more common answers. Especially as we age, we want to train smarter, not harder. Sometimes that includes more rest, more strength training, more preparatory work, more awareness, and more progressive builds to get there.

Tips When Recovering From Injury

1. Professional assessment
2. Modified activity
3. Corrective exercise focus
4. Cross-training
5. Gradual and progressive return to volume, intensity, load, and velocity
6. Maintenance

Walking Tips When Returning From Injury

1. Begin with good posture and walking technique.
2. Walk slower.
3. Take smaller steps.
4. Walk for shorter periods of time.
5. Warm up and cool down.
6. Seek treatment.

Injury Prevention Strategies

Focus on a few key strategies to prevent injuries. After having helped a number of individuals recover from injury, it's clear that prevention is key. Recovering from injury can be a very frustrating and long process. Prevention, intervention, correction, and maintenance will keep us on track.

First, you'll want to ensure that you're warming up and cooling down properly (chapter 6). Include specific preparatory work after warming up to prime, activate, and bring awareness to certain areas, especially if you know you've had issues with an injury in the past. During your walks, focus on proper posture and technique (chapter 5).

Another important injury prevention element is sticking to progressive overload principles. Because walking is a fairly accessible, convenient, and easy form of movement, it can be easy to overdo it. Start with a base that you know is comfortable and doable for your body. Increase the volume and intensity slowly, aiming for a 10 percent increase in distance each week and adding higher-intensity intervals slowly. Performing smaller volumes at more frequent intensities can help to more rapidly adapt while modulating stress. Splitting workouts up throughout the day is an option to help attenuate stress. Four 30-minute walks may be easier to tolerate than two 60-minute walks over a week-long period. Just as splitting or spreading walks out throughout the day may help us adapt and recover, a slow progressive build will allow our bodies to adapt to more volume and intensity more readily and with more support.

A short cool-down and stretch after your walk will start the recovery process and help your body feel more comfortable. Fitting strength and corrective exercises in will help you build a more resilient and balanced system. Ask for help when you're stuck, and address pains and discomforts quickly to avoid worsening symptoms and lengthy recoveries.

Just as we adapt and progress in our own unique way, our recovery is also distinct and individual. Every one of us will progress and recover at differing levels. Perhaps this is why we don't have strong evidence surrounding exercise and recovery strategies, because the effectiveness of certain strategies is unique to each person. We also need to consider our mental and emotional states, activities of daily living, and our total available bandwidth for all that life demands, because it will all play a role in the body's ability to push and recover.

Injury Prevention Strategies

1. Warm-up
2. Preparatory work and corrective exercise
3. Proper walking form
4. Progressive overload
5. Cool-down and mobility work
6. Maintenance

Recovery

We are only as strong as what we can essentially recover from. Recovering from our workouts will help us to build strength, stamina, stability, sustainability, and repeatability. Recovering from your workouts promotes healing and allows you to return to exercise faster and with more comfort. Many of our systems are built-in repair phases (e.g., rest and sleep), and it is important to cool down, rest, and recover. Resting and actively recovering allows our bodies to restore, recuperate, repair, and build the strength and capacity required to perform the same activity and more the next time we're physically active. All gains are made during the recovery phase. We outline specific recovery tips and strategies next.

Active Recovery

Exercise can make us feel fatigued, and in some cases, sore and achy. Although movement is critical for overall health and fitness, we also need to recover well from our movement so that we are prepared for our next bout of activity. The term *active recovery* refers to performing a lower-intensity exercise for a short duration following a period of higher-intensity exercise to help improve overall recovery. A few minutes of slower-paced walking at the end of our moderate to vigorous walk, for example, can help you recover faster and reduce the likelihood of muscle tears and pain. Performing lower-intensity activity between intervals or on rest or off days is also active recovery. A 2018 study found that the enhanced blood flow in muscle tissue from active recovery helped to remove metabolic waste and may contribute to reduced muscle tearing and pain (Dupuy et al. 2018).

We are only able to perform and push our hardest if we can recover from our last workout. We can push harder when we are well rested. Although we often want to finish up and head back to our day, spending a few purposeful minutes slowing down is advantageous.

Sleep

We simply can't discount the importance of quality sleep to aid in our overall recovery. A good night's sleep will do wonders to restore and refresh bodies and brains. Sleep is a key component to recovery that is often overlooked. Doing what you can to ensure optimal sleep assists in recovery and overall health. Make your room dark, avoid screens before bed, eat well throughout the day, avoid caffeine and stimulants later in the day, and include some downregulation strategies before bed through meditation, deep breathing, or active relaxation. Seek professional help if you struggle with sleep quantity and quality.

Nutrition and Hydration

We touched on the importance of nutrition and hydration in chapter 3. Ensuring we are well fueled and well hydrated before and after workouts means we have the available nutrients, building blocks, and foundation required to recover from all of our activities.

Proper Warm-Up and Cool-Down

We've dedicated an entire chapter to warm-ups and cool-downs, and it warrants repeating here. There's immense value in priming and cooling down to help you perform at your best and recover well. Warming up and cooling down properly will play a key role in overall recovery (see chapter 6).

Seeking Therapies

When we opened our studio and clinic in 2011, including complementary therapies (e.g., Massage therapy, Physiotherapy, etc.) was on the top of our list. We loved the idea of a multidisciplinary approach where our clients could come to receive quality coaching and care in many forms, through massage therapy, physiotherapy, or athletic therapy in conjunction with coaching services. It made sense from a holistic perspective, and we know the importance of ongoing therapy for overall health. Multidisciplinary approaches including physical therapy provide long-term improvements in pain and functional status of patients with nonspecific chronic low back pain (Sahin et al. 2017). In addition, foam rolling, stretching, self-massage, and other forms of myofascial release can boost your recovery. A 2019 study found that foam rolling was useful in reducing delayed onset of muscle soreness (DOMS) after high-intensity interval training (Laffaye et al. 2019). Some studies have found that runners had improved recovery when using massage therapy after exercise versus a control group (Duñabeitia et al. 2022). Massage therapy helps to reduce cortisol levels (stress hormones) and increase dopamine and serotonin (happy hormones) (Field et al. 2005). If you feel better with the treatments (self-administered or not), it's helpful. If it's within your means and you feel rejuvenated, using therapy at intervals that work for you can assist with an overall sense of well-being, even if they won't specifically assist in postexercise recovery.

Corrective Exercise, Strength, and Maintenance

In chapter 9, we'll discuss the importance of building strength and muscle mass in more detail. Building and maintaining muscle mass as we age helps to prevent sarcopenia; support our metabolic health, bone health, and cardiovascular health; and promote overall strength, longevity, and stability. An important element of injury prevention is strength, stability, and clean movement mechanics. Correcting patterns, imbalances, weaknesses, or cracks in our foundations will help increase our thresholds so that we can withstand more volumes, intensities, velocities, and loads without breaking down, pain, discomfort, or injury. Staying on top of our corrective exercise and strength training regimes is a good prevention and recovery strategy.

Rest

Rest plays a key role in overall recovery. When we continually exercise and break things down, we don't have ample opportunities to rebuild and regenerate. Take a look at your big-picture week, month, or year to periodize and ensure you have balanced workouts with walking, strength, and cross-training. Build in rest days to ensure optimal recovery. Make time for lower-intensity days and stretching and mobility work. Pay attention to how you feel. If your body feels more fatigued than usual, you're waking up with an elevated heart rate, you're feeling achy and having a hard time getting motivated to exercise, or you suspect relative energy deficiency in sport (RED-S), consult with a medical professional and add in more rest days.

This chapter has provided some ideas on how to recover, bridge the gap back to your usual routine, and remain active while you heal from an injury. In chapter 9, we'll provide numerous examples of how to strengthen various muscle groups. Strengthening is an excellent way to build tissue resilience, prevent injuries, increase longevity, and improve overall health and wellness.

CHAPTER 9

Strength Training for Walkers

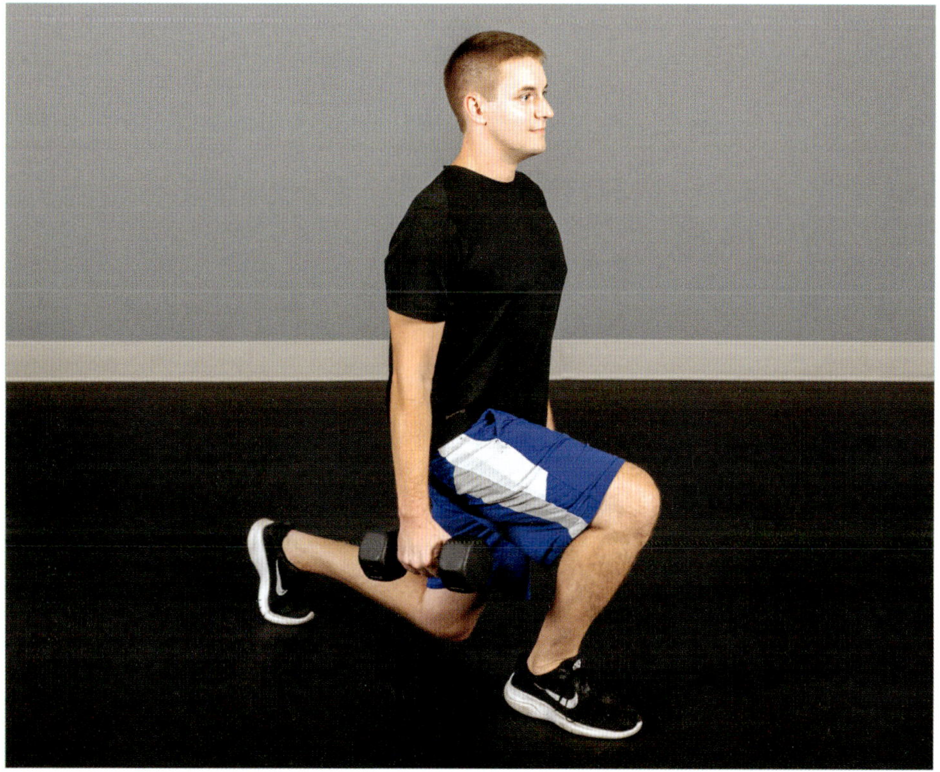

This chapter is likely the most important chapter to read and implement. Strength training is critical for every person. For walkers, strength training is arguably the most complementary form of activity. Being strong reduces the risk of injuries, adds more propulsion to walking, improves posture and bone density, increases metabolism, and prevents sarcopenia as we age. Including some form of strength training in your overall programming is important in terms of longevity, strength, metabolic health, disease prevention, muscle preservation, bone health, power, balance, stability, physical performance, comfort, movement control, cognitive health, independence, and more. Walking alone is not sufficient from an exercise perspective. Strength training not only helps me feel strong and able but also gives me confidence because I know I am doing everything possible to live comfortably, independently, and productively as I age. I want to be able to open jars, sit and stand with ease, lift heavy objects without difficulty, carry grandchildren around, and walk as much as I would like in my 60s, 70s, 80s, and beyond. The investment starts now.

Adults will lose 3 to 8 percent of muscle mass per decade along with a reduction in metabolic rate and an increase in fat accumulation (Westcott 2012). Many of our national guidelines recommend strength training in addition to aerobic training to achieve optimal health. The Canadian Society for Exercise Physiology (2021) recommends that Canadians obtain at least 150 minutes of moderate to vigorous physical activity, plus at least two muscle-strengthening sessions using major muscle groups weekly. Americans ideally should be obtaining 150 to 300 minutes a week of moderate-intensity or 150 minutes of vigorous-intensity aerobic activity weekly as well as muscle-strengthening activities of moderate or greater intensity that involve all major muscle groups on two or more days a week (U.S. Department of Health and Human Services 2018). Europe and many other countries have similar guidelines, with some adding balance training for adults over the age of 65 to assist in fall prevention (European Union 2008). In essence, exercise is important and highly recommended to keep our populations healthy. Yet, in 2020 studies, only 43.9 percent of Canadians and 24.2 percent of Americans met these national guidelines regularly (Statistics Canada 2021; National Center for Health Statistics 2020).

The benefits of strength training are widely studied and numerous. Strength training is medicine (Westcott 2012). People who strength train are less likely to die than those who don't (Momma 2022). According to the meta-analysis by Momma (2022), those who performed 30 to 60 minutes of strength training weekly had a 10 to 20 percent lower risk of cancer, heart disease, and death from all causes. Strength training includes some of the following benefits:

- Increased strength (Maestroni et al. 2020)
- Improved heart health (MacDonald et al. 2016)
- Improved metabolic health (Lee et al. 2017; Shiroma et al. 2017)
- Decreased risk of injury (Suchomel et al. 2018; Lauersen et al. 2018)
- Decreased risk of falls (Sherrington et al. 2019)
- Stronger bones (Mosti et al. 2014; Beck et al. 2017)
- Improved brain health and mental health (Gordon et al. 2017)
- Improved blood sugar management and decreased risk of type 2 diabetes (Shiroma et al. 2017)
- Decreased visceral fat (the dangerous fat that surrounds your organs) (Yarizadeh et al. 2021)

- Correction of muscle imbalances (Gioftsidou et al. 2008)
- Better quality of life (Kekäläinen et al. 2018)

Strength training helps us to reduce the risk of disease and live longer with higher functionality and quality of life. For those with type 2 diabetes, strength training is a more effective treatment than aerobic training alone (Kobayashi et al. 2023). Strength training allows us to have more endurance, strength, power, and mobility. Even the founder of aerobics, Ken Cooper, now states, "As you grow older, the need to do strength training becomes increasingly important to help you [slow] the loss of muscle and bone mass" (Cooper 1999).

Strength training can be done with minimal equipment. As you get stronger, you can slowly invest in more pieces (or a gym membership). Dumbbells, barbells, kettlebells, or other heavy objects can be used. Bands and our own body weight can be appropriate tools as well.

Foundation

In this section you will find a list of essential exercises to add into your overall fitness plan, along with options for various fitness levels. These exercises will help to improve overall strength and stability. The emphasis is on general strength, single-leg stability (key for walkers), core stability, and posture.

Aim to perform two or three sets of 8 to 10 repetitions for each exercise (unless otherwise indicated), working to fatigue. The dynamic warm-up drills from chapter 6 can be used as movement preparation for the strength exercises, and the stretches from chapter 6 can be used after a workout. These exercises should not be the only strength exercises you would perform, because adding in more progressive challenges will be key for strength gains, but they serve as a starting point and options for complementing your walks. Aim to change your exercise programming every 4 to 10 weeks by varying the exercises, sets, repetitions, load, and tempo.

Order of Events

1. Dynamic, purposeful warm-up drills (chapter 6): 3 to 5 minutes
2. Strength train (2 or 3 sets of 8 to 10 repetitions): 6 to 8 exercises, major muscles
3. Postworkout stretch (chapter 6): 3 to 5 minutes

BIRD DOG

The bird dog is a commonly prescribed back exercise. It can be a great tool to help build cylinder control, multifidus and back recruitment, and core connections. As we engage our core and move our limbs, we'll build good opposite limb coordination, which is seen in walking. It's important to move slowly and with control, while keeping the back straight and still as you move the arms and legs. Moving quickly and with excessive lumbar motion takes away from the back stabilizing benefits. Feedback tools like balls or blocks placed on the low back while performing the bird dog can really help us to feel the stability here. Place a ball or block on the low back and try to do the exercise without it falling off. This will require a greater amount of concentration and stabilization.

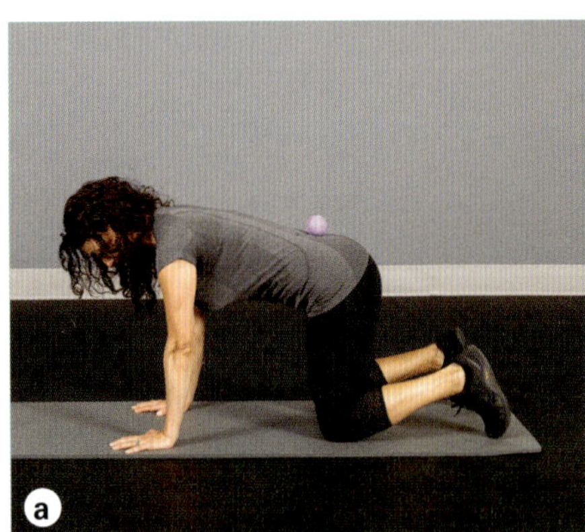

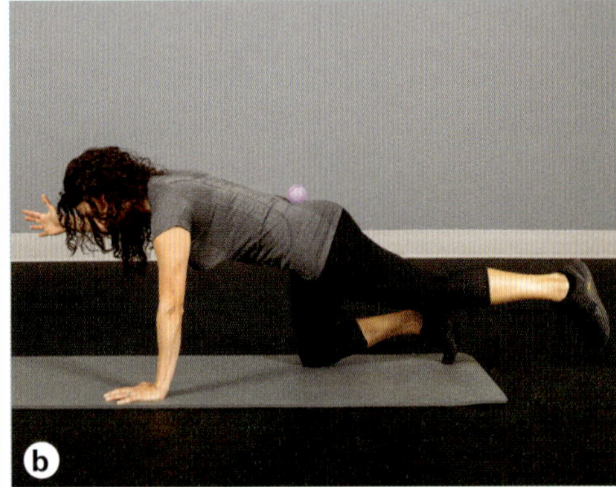

Instructions

Start on all fours (in a quadruped position) with your hands placed under your shoulders and your knees under your hips. Place a ball or block on the low back and aim to keep it still. Spread your fingers wide and push your hands into the ground to prevent sinking into your shoulder blades. Bring your shoulders away from your ears and aim to engage your lats by thinking of spinning or rotating the wrists out (without moving them) *(a)*. Engage your core, exhale, and extend one arm and opposite leg while keeping your back straight *(b)*. Alternate sides while maintaining a slow tempo with control and stability.

Variations

If the ball or block on the back is challenging for you, start without it and slowly work your way up. Set up in the standard bird dog position *(c)* and start by extending your leg and keeping it on the floor as you glide it in and switch sides *(d)*. Once you feel comfortable with that variation, add a shoulder tap by picking up the opposite hand and tapping the shoulder. From there, you can add a leg lift and work toward adding the full arm extension.

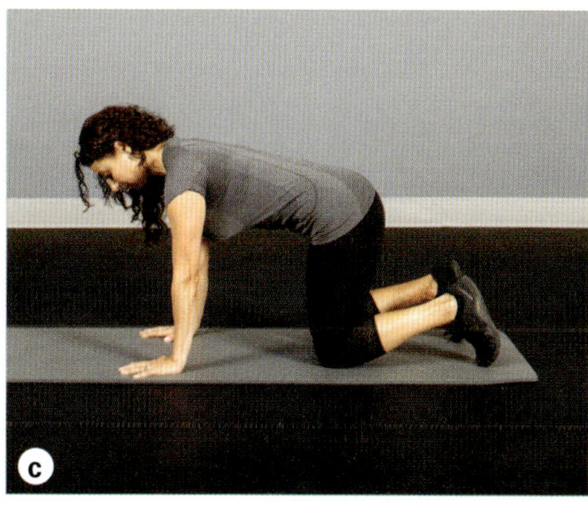
c

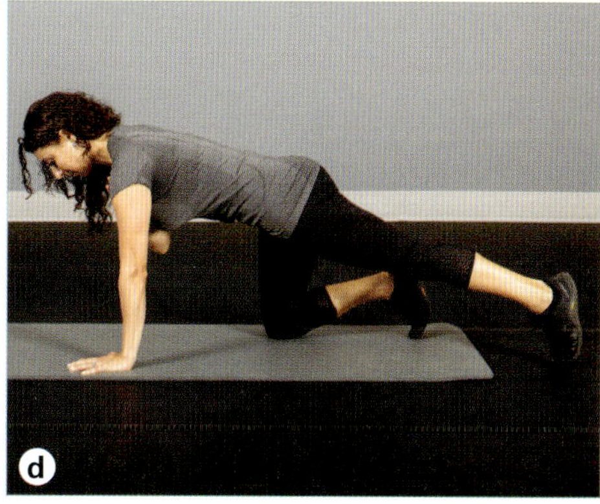
d

For a more challenging bird dog variation, add a band around your foot and hold it with the opposite hand *(e)*. Extend your arm and leg with the added challenge of the band *(f)*. Switch sides after the desired number of repetitions.

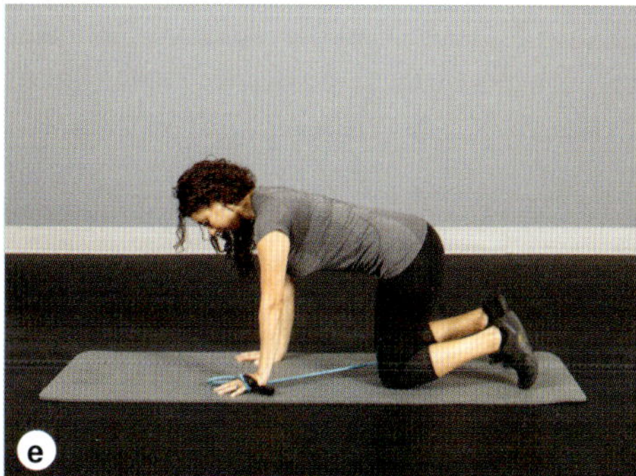
e

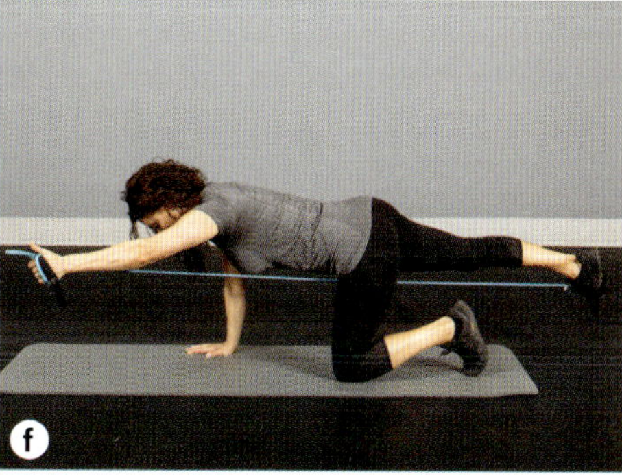
f

Alternatively, bring your bird dog to an upright position, place your hands on a chair or stability ball, and press into the chair or ball *(g)*. Extend the arm and leg while still maintaining the straight back alignment *(h)*. Exhale and engage the core to extend and alternate sides.

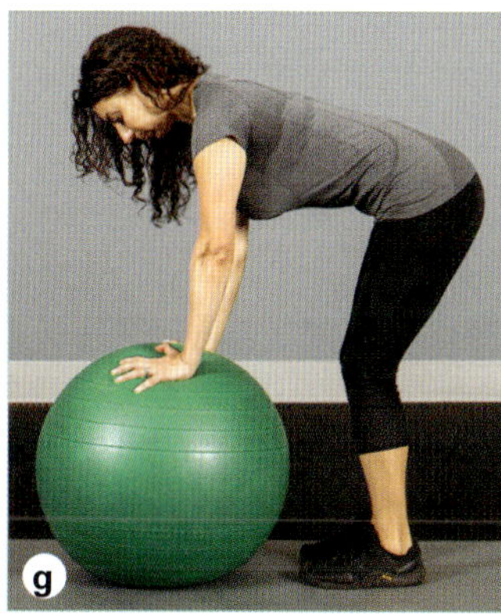
g

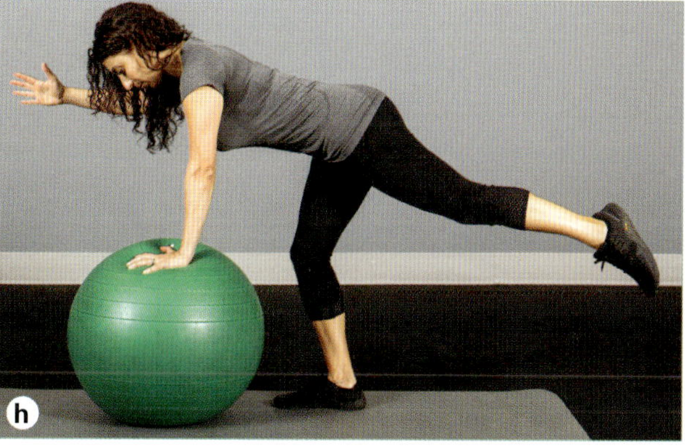
h

DUMBBELL STANDING REAR GLIDE

The rear glide is a great exercise to help build single-leg stability. I learned this exercise from Scott and Jaime Livingston years ago and have implemented variations of it in many of my clients' programs as well as my own with much success. Jaime Sochasky Livingston, Certified Athletic Therapist and cofounder of Neuro Reconditioning and the educational company ReconditioningHQ.com, shares her take on this exercise: "Effective ambulation (walking) requires, with each step, the ability to stack the body well over a single lower limb and foot, while moving the opposite leg, without compromising the standing-foot connection and pressure, center-of-gravity positioning, or the midline orientation of the pelvis and spine to each other. The rear glide exercise allows you to build on this vital 'single-leg pillar' posture capacity while developing more efficient dissociative movement with the opposite 'swing' leg."

The goal of the exercise is to maintain a stable and stacked "pillar" posture on the standing leg while moving the opposite leg (similar to walking, in a sense), working the capacity to keep a solid standing-foot position, a body center-of-gravity position, as well as a stable pelvis and spine. "A pillar position is when the foot, shin, and thigh are in a neutral alignment stacked on top of each other with a level pelvis and tall spine posture in the torso. While the lower limb and nervous system require the coordination of many muscles to achieve this task, muscles of interest involved in this task are those involved in maintaining upright posture, for example, the gluteus medius, gluteus maximus, and other hip and core stabilizers" shares Sochasky Livingston.

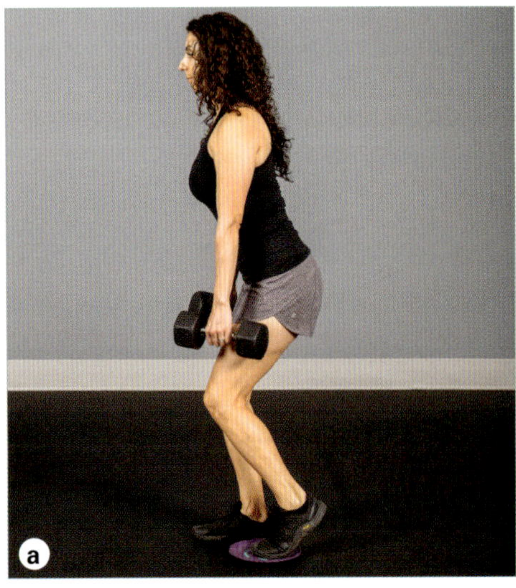

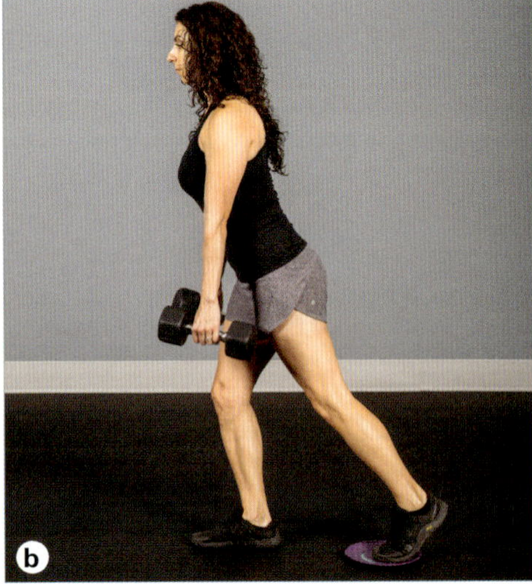

Instructions

While standing, bend both knees slightly and shift your weight from two feet to one foot to create and maintain a good foot connection and pressure into the ground. Then, slightly hinge your hips so that your upper body and torso tip to lean forward slightly into a similar angle to that of your shins *(a)*. Keep the weight in your standing midfoot area and resist keeping the pressure backward onto your heel. With your arms by your sides, slowly glide the swing leg straight back to bring it alongside your standing heel *(b)*. There should be very little pressure into the ground from the moving leg (just enough to help with balance and stability)—the pressure control and position of the standing foot and leg should be the focus in this task. Continue gliding the swing-leg foot back and forth while the standing leg is in the pillar position with the knee bent and hip hinged. You can glide the swing foot in sock feet on smooth flooring or place a towel or disk under your gliding foot. "The focus should remain on maintaining the midfoot pressure of the standing-leg foot and a stacked pillar position while breathing calmly throughout the movement. You may feel you are working harder than you expect and, if so, probably doing it well. If you're feeling discomfort, you can try to reduce or even stop the motion of the swing leg or adjust where the pressure is on the stance-leg foot," shares Sochasky Livingston.

Variations

For an easier variation, try holding on to a wall or broomstick for more support *(c-d)*. For more of a challenge, aim to hold dumbbells or kettlebells in each of your hands. For a greater balance challenge, aim to hover the moving foot off the floor.

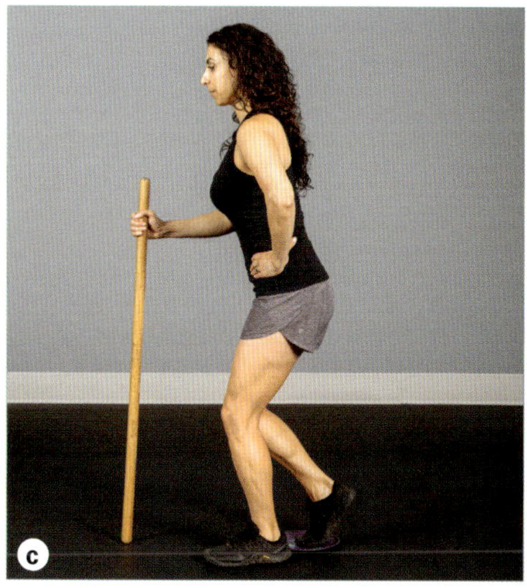
c

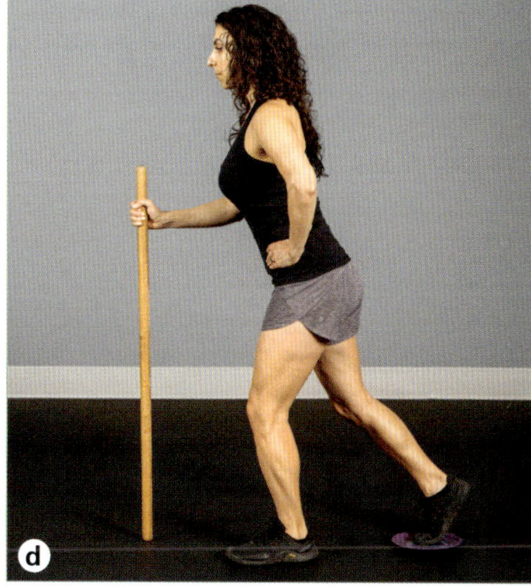
d

SPLIT SQUAT

The split squat is an excellent functional and purposeful exercise to build lower body strength. It's important to include exercises and challenges that mimic our day-to-day lives, especially as we age, and squatting is one of those exercises. It's essential to maintain the strength to sit and stand up from varying surfaces with comfort and ease.

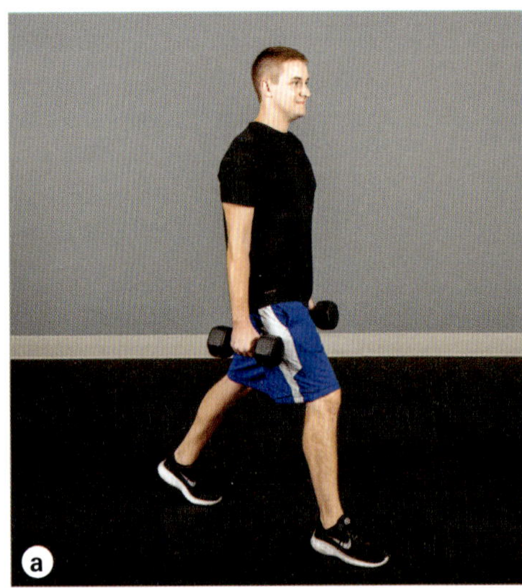

a

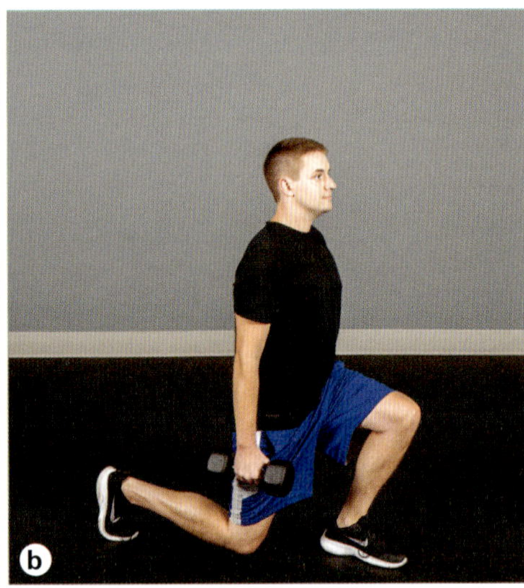

b

Instructions

Start by standing with your feet about hip-width apart and take a large step backward with your back heel elevated *(a)*. You'll end up sharing the weight between your front foot and back toes (your back heel is off the ground). Aim to put 70 percent of your body weight in the front foot. Bend both knees, aiming to create 90-degree angles with each leg *(b)*. Keep your back straight (with a slight forward lean) and come back up to your start position. Once you're comfortable with the pattern, hold weights in each hand.

Variations

Regress the split squat by starting with a squat. Stand tall with your feet shoulder-width apart (or slightly wider if more comfortable) *(c)*. Your feet can be turned out slightly if this feels more natural for you. Begin by bending your knees and hinging your hips, aiming to have your spine and shins parallel to each other *(d)*. Keep the back straight and the chest open. Go as deep as possible without having the tailbone tuck under. Press through the feet to come up.

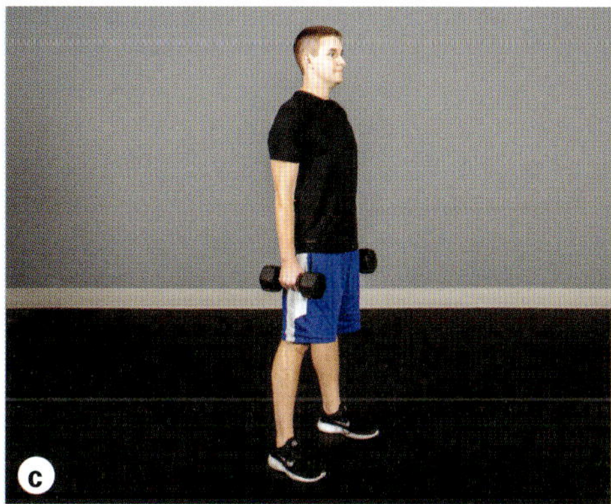
c

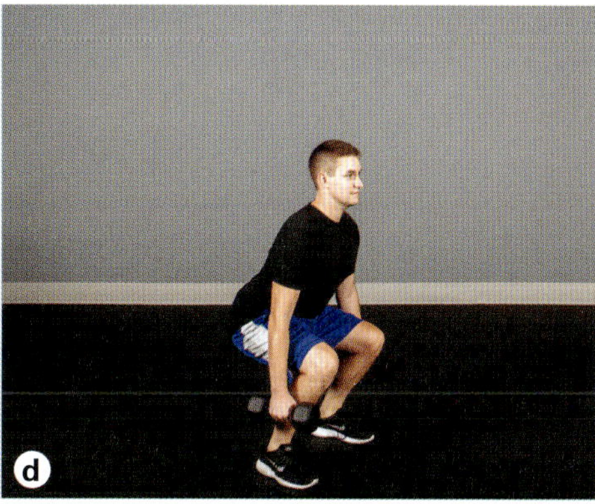
d

For a more challenging variation, try an alternating reverse lunge. Start by standing tall *(e)* and step back into a lunge position (two 90-degree angles with the legs) *(f)*. Press through the front foot to come back to your standing position. Repeat on the other side.

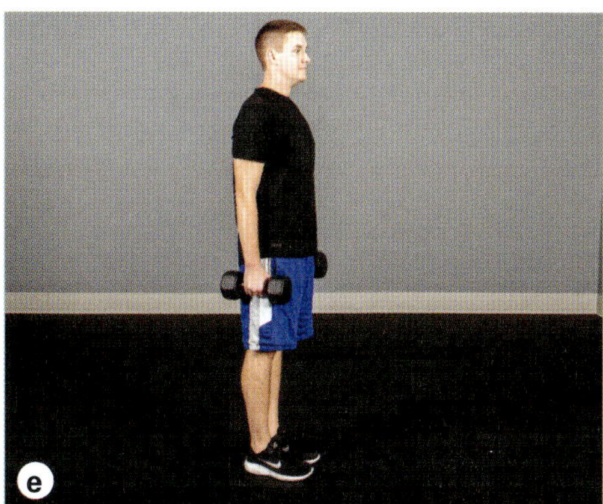
e

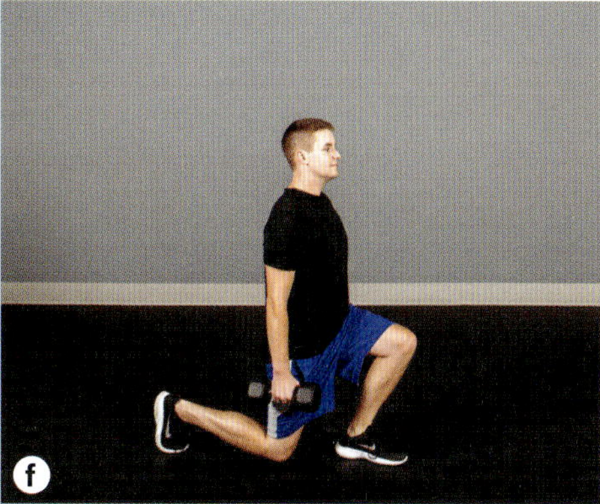
f

STANDING BAND ROW

When walking briskly, the backward arm drive becomes a key element, and having the comfort and full range with this pattern is helpful. Although we are using more momentum than strength when walking, strong back muscles assist a multitude of elements like posture, pulling, balancing out strong upper body anterior muscles, back support, injury prevention, and comfort, among other things.

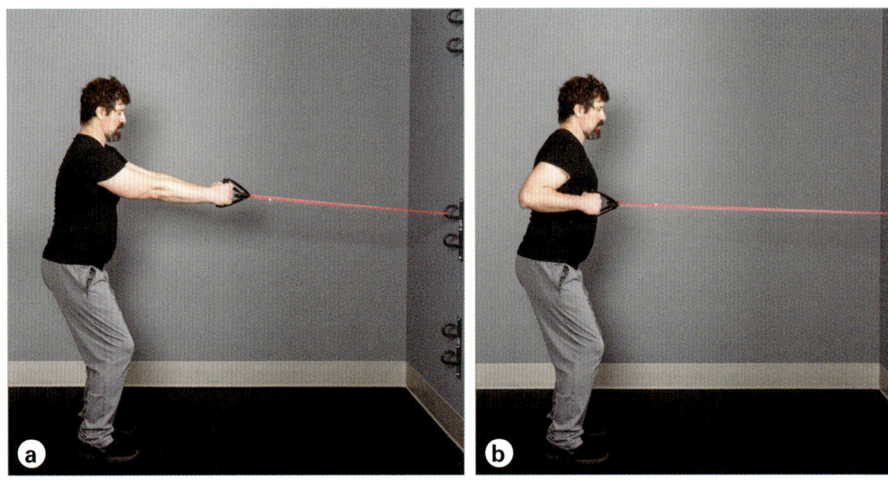

Instructions

Place a band around a secure object positioned at chest height (a post, solid railing, exercise machine, or door anchor would work well). Stand tall and hold one end of the band in each hand. Bend your knees slightly, lean forward slightly, and keep your chest open and back straight *(a)*. Pull the band in toward you, keeping your forearms parallel to the floor and your palms facing inward as you bring your elbows back *(b)*. Try not to roll the shoulders inward; keep them in an open position as you row. Slowly straighten the arms.

Variations

For an easier variation, start with just your arms (no band) to perfect the pattern, and progress to a light band.

For a more challenging variation, use a heavier band. Or try the bent-over row variation by holding a dumbbell in each hand, bending your knees, and hinging your hips while keeping your back straight. Lean forward with a straight back and maintain a good connection with the feet pressing into the ground. The arms start by hanging down by your sides *(c)*. Bring the dumbbells back slightly and row, keeping the dumbbells parallel to the floor as you bring them up to just below your chest *(d)*. Keep the shoulders down away from the ears as you row and focus on pulling with the back.

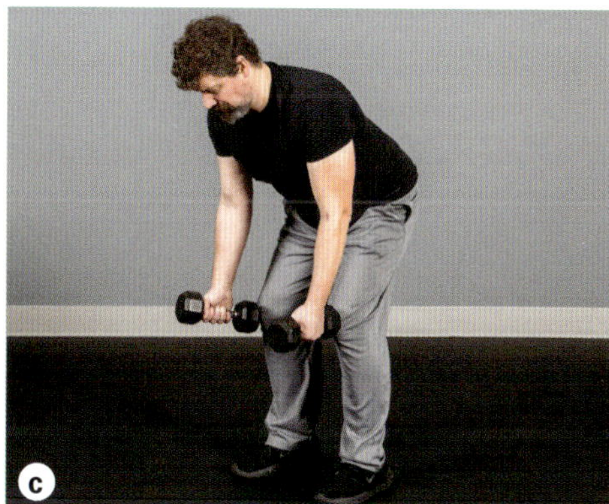

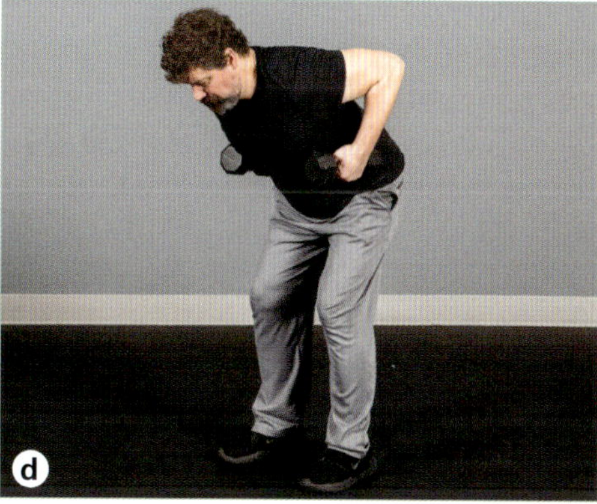

Using one arm at a time for the band row *(e)* or bent-over row option *(f)* can increase the overall challenge.

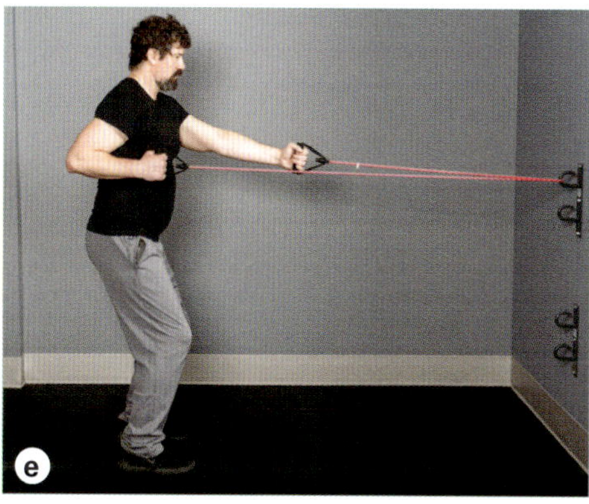

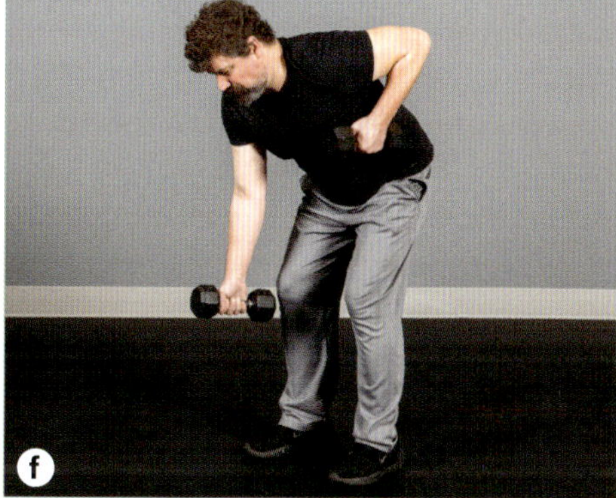

SINGLE-LEG KICKSTAND DEADLIFT

The deadlift is a key movement pattern for our day-to-day lives. Understanding how to hinge properly protects our backs and increases our strength and comfort when lifting objects off the floor. The deadlift also builds strength in the posterior chain, improves our mechanics surrounding lifting, and improves balance in the body. Strong hip and leg muscles help to power our walks. We'll be focusing on the Romanian deadlift (RDL) variation or stiff-legged variation because it tends to be a bit easier to focus on hinging one area (hips) versus three (hips, knees, and ankles) and will put a greater emphasis on the posterior chain.

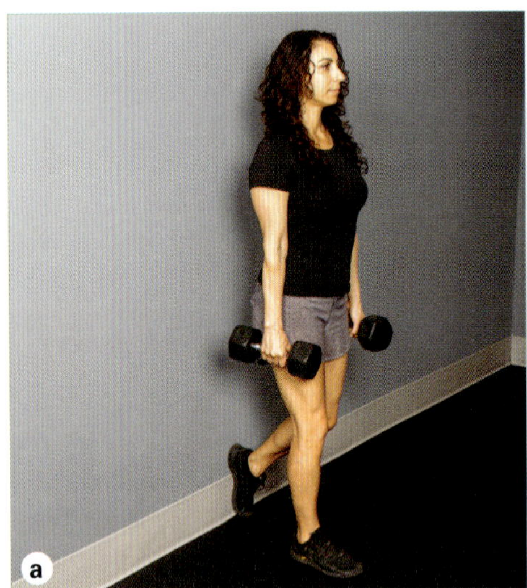

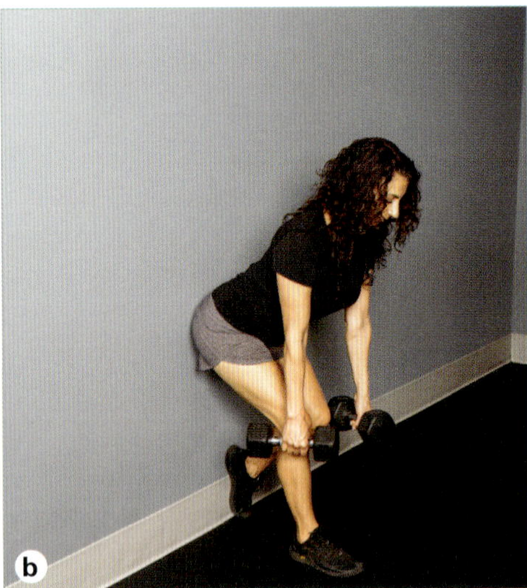

Instructions

We can bias one side by moving into a kickstand position. Stand facing away from a wall, and place one foot about 12 inches (or 30 cm) away from the wall. Place the other foot against the wall with the heel up the wall and the toes on the floor. Put the weight on the front, standing leg *(a)*. Hinge your hips and try to touch your hips against the wall behind you while keeping your back straight *(b)*. Your hands should not drop much farther than your knees. Return to your start position by pressing down into the feet (think of a foot tripod—heel, ball of the foot, and outer edge of the foot). Your hips and shoulders move in tandem. When your hips hit the wall, stop moving your shoulders. Additional shoulder and back movement beyond this point will load more of the lumbar spine. Perform all your repetitions on one side before switching sides.

Variations

To regress, start with the bilateral RDL. Begin by standing tall with a slight bend in the knees *(c)*. Open the chest and aim to keep your back straight throughout. Hinge your hips back, thinking of bringing your sit bones to the wall behind you and continuing this hip-hinging motion *(d)*. Your arms will follow the line of the thighs. Try not to reach your arms forward and lean forward; think of moving your hips back instead. Hold dumbbells for an increased challenge.

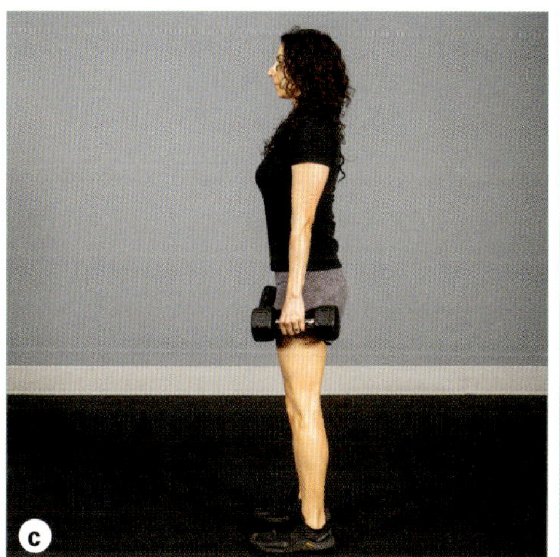
c

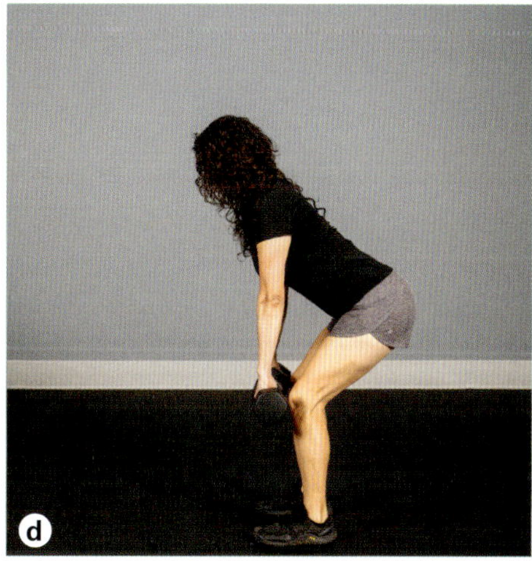
d

Once you've mastered the RDL, try the single-leg variation. In the single-leg variation, stand on one leg and kick the other leg behind you with the foot off the floor *(e)*. Begin hinging by bringing your back leg high to keep the pelvis level as you hinge forward *(f)*.

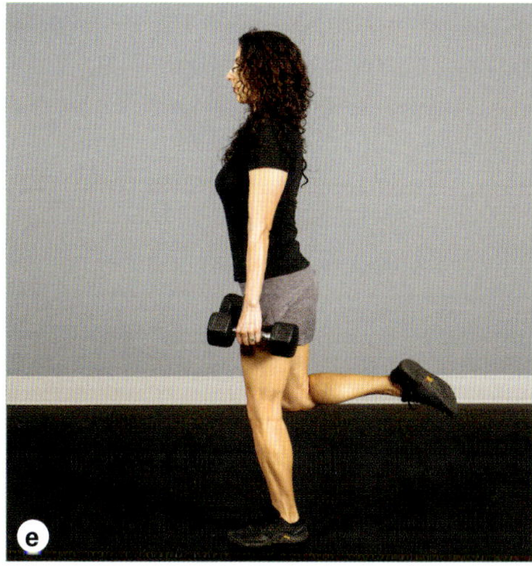
e

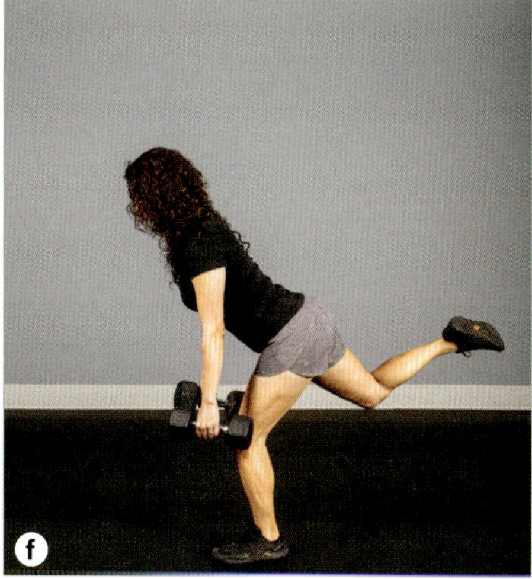
f

DUMBBELL SIDE-LYING REAR DELT RAISE

This exercise strengthens the posterior deltoid. This muscle works to externally rotate the shoulder, which will help us to walk with better posture and shoulder positioning as the shoulders tend to round inward. The posterior deltoid also plays a role in humeral (or arm) extension. The backward arm drive helps to propel us forward. Strengthening these muscles improves our posture and backward arm drive during our walks.

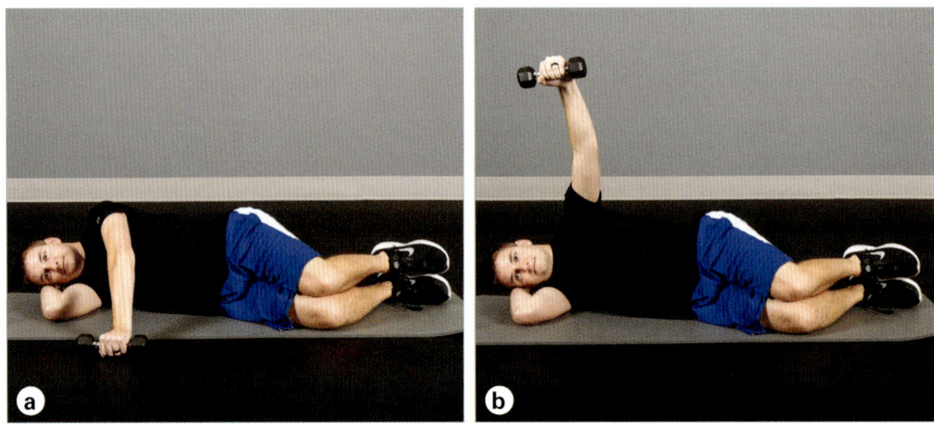

Instructions

Lie on your side with your knees bent and the bottom arm bent to support your head. Hold a light dumbbell in the top hand and extend your arm straight out from your shoulder *(a)*. Place a slight bend in the arm with the elbow pointing up to the ceiling. Maintain that fixed arm position as you raise the arm up, stopping just before parallel to the wall *(b)*, and return to your start position without bending or extending your elbow. Slowly increase the weight as you become more comfortable.

Variations

For a greater challenge, try starting on a higher surface such as a bench, step, or couch, and aim to move through a fuller range of motion as you lower the weight toward the floor to start *(c-d)*.

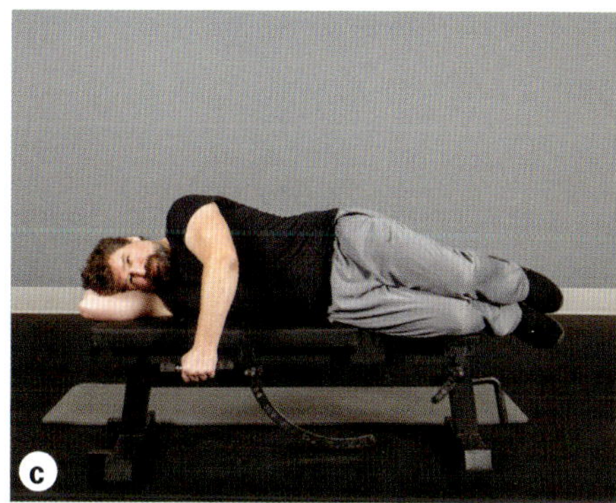

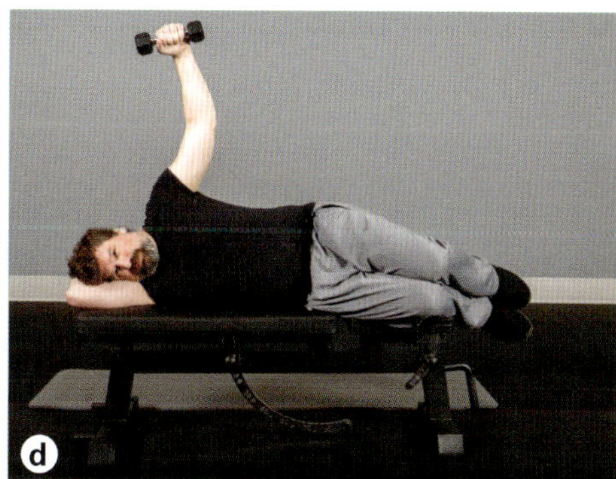

Alternatively, this exercise can be done from a standing position. Bent-over rear flies can be done by hinging forward while keeping a straight back position with your knees bent. Hold the weights in each hand, place a small bend in each arm, and allow the hands to be positioned under the shoulders and in front of the knees *(e)*. Maintain that small bend as you raise your arms out to the sides, stopping just before your arms reach parallel to the floor *(f)*. Slowly return to the start position.

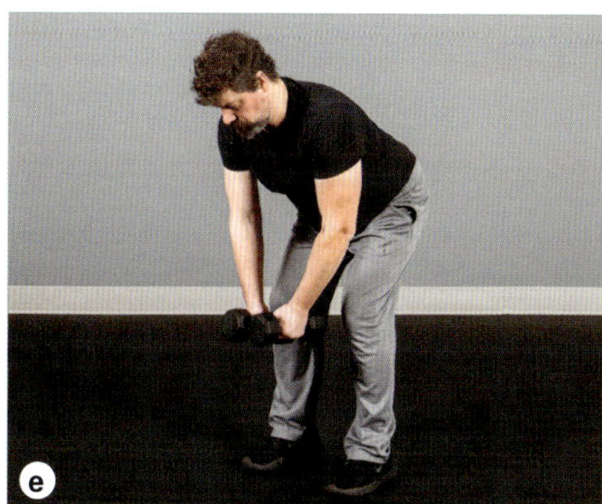

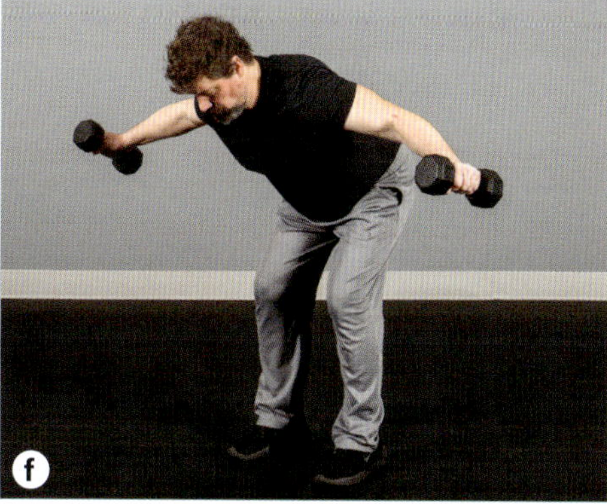

PALLOF PRESS

The Pallof press using a band or cable machine is a great standing core variation. As walkers, it's important to include several standing strength and core challenges that closely mimic our activity. Challenging our core muscles in an upright position can help with the functional crossover to walking.

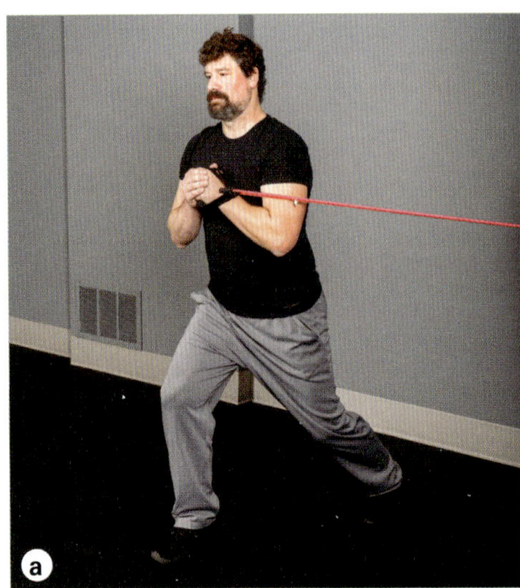

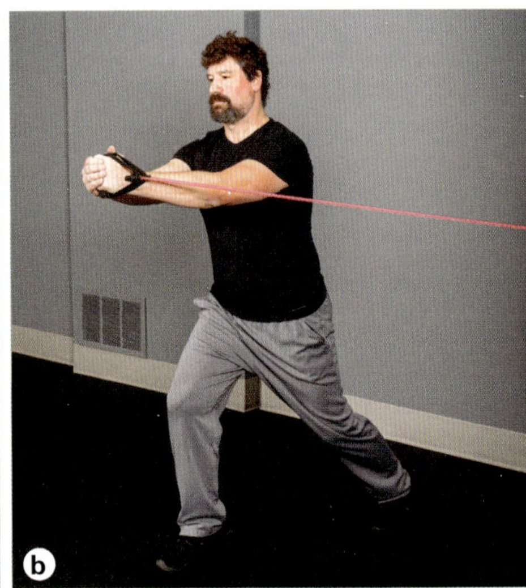

Instructions

Attach a band around a secure object (e.g., post, railing, door anchor, exercise machine) and hold the band in both hands at chest level. Stand 90 degrees from your anchor so that one side of the body is closest to the anchor, with your feet in a split position, both knees slightly bent, your outside leg forward, and your back heel up *(a)*. The majority of the weight is on the front foot, and the foot is active and grounded. Lean forward slightly, think of engaging your core, and exhale to press the arms straight forward, keeping your hands at the same level of the chest and centered *(b)*. Hold the arm-extended position for a second (or longer) before returning to your start position.

Variations

You can make the Pallof press easier by standing in a bilateral stance with both feet side by side and the knees slightly bent *(c-d)*.

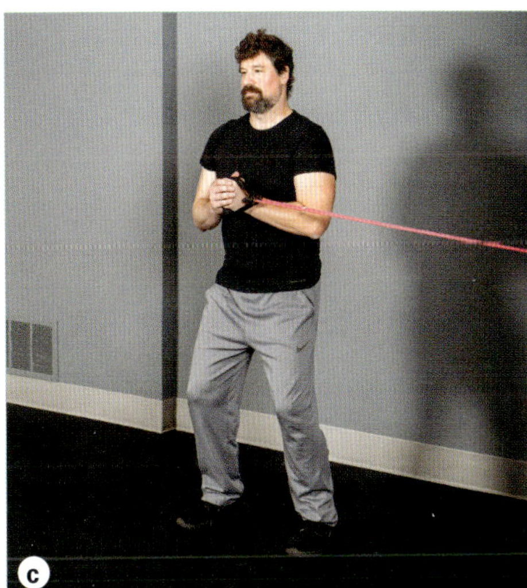

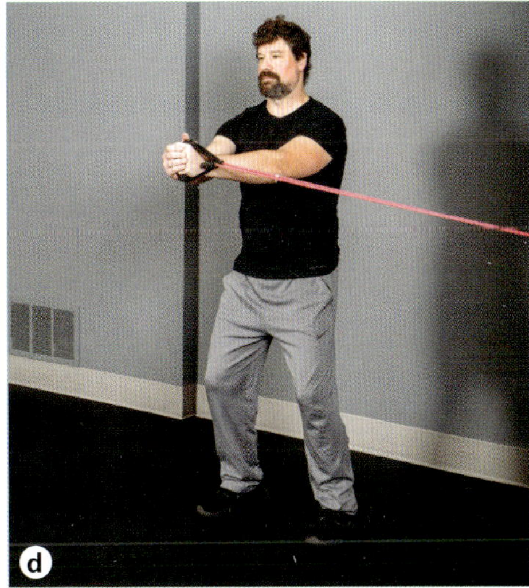

For a greater challenge, stand farther away from your anchor point or use a stronger resistance of band or cable machine as resistance.

DYING BUG

This exercise (sometimes referred to as *dead bug*) is one that focuses on challenging the core while moving the arms and legs. The movement engages opposite limbs (e.g., right arm, left leg movement), similar to a walking pattern. Think of a core connection and contraction during the exercise; however, we don't want to grip our core muscles while we're walking (see Core Gripping and Glute Gripping).

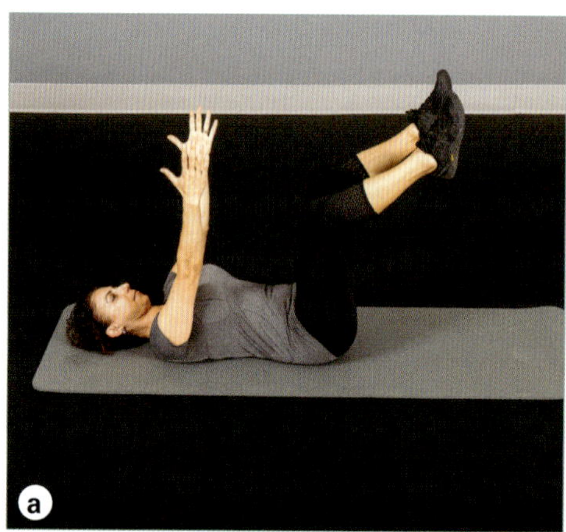

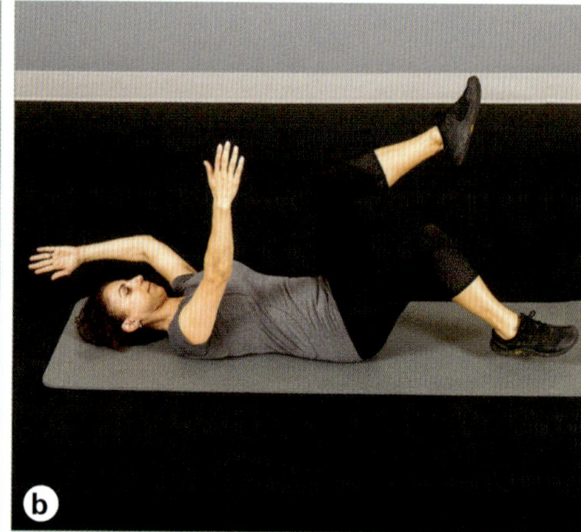

Instructions

Start by lying on your back with your arms extended toward the ceiling and your legs bent at 90 degrees *(a)*. Tuck your chin in so your head, neck, and back are aligned. Ensure your ribs are aligned with your hips, as we don't want our ribs flaring upward. Feel the low ribs making contact with the floor from the back. Begin by engaging the core, exhale, and think of a belt-tightening sensation; imagine your hip bones closing and hug the ribs closer together from the front. You can place your hand on your abdomen to feel your core, aiming to keep your belly pulled away from your hand. Extend one arm and the opposite leg toward the ground while keeping the abdominals held in and the low ribs connected to the ground *(b)*. Inhale to return to your start position and repeat on the other side. Aim to contract the core just enough to support the weight of the legs and movement (a core-contracting strategy that is too strong may place additional pressure on the back and core by increasing intra-abdominal pressure).

Variations

For an easier variation (and a great starting point), try moving just the legs. Keep the hands on the belly, and exhale and engage the core to lower one leg at a time *(c-d)*.

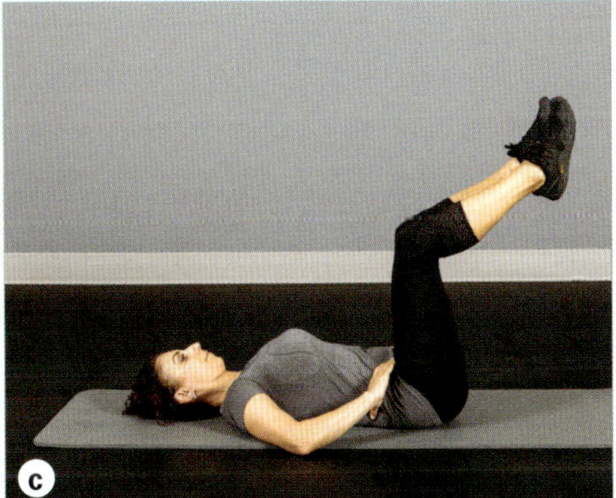
c

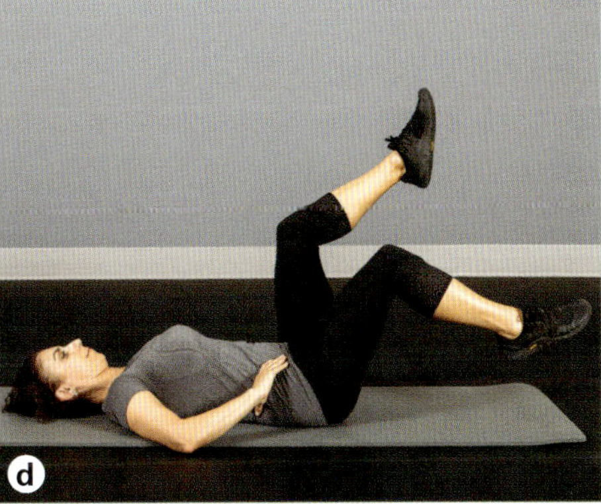
d

If that feels too challenging and you're noticing the belly pushing upward, start with both feet on the floor and lift one leg at a time *(e-f)*. March slowly and aim to keep your hips stable as you switch sides.

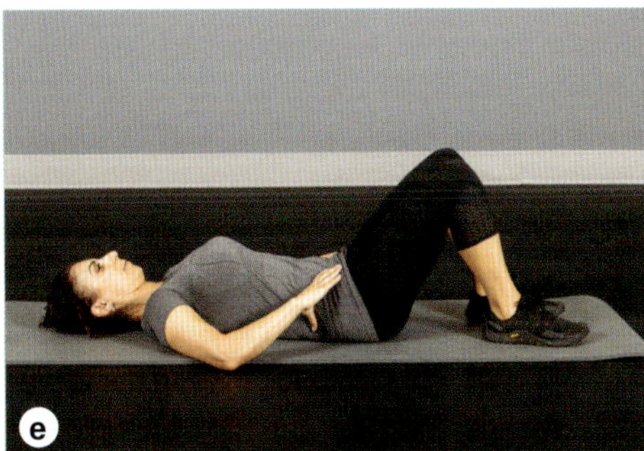
e

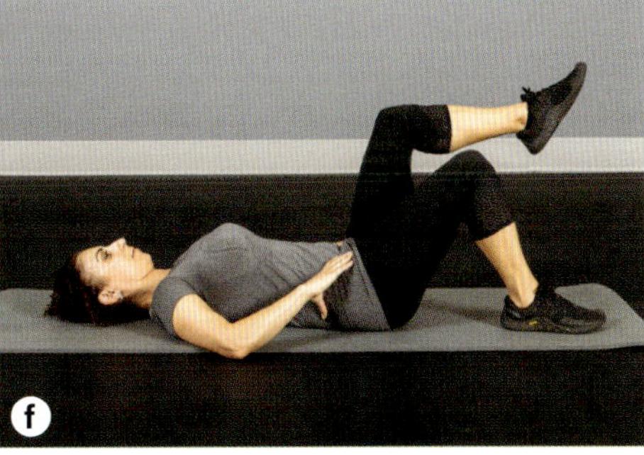
f

For a more challenging variation, press one hand into the opposite thigh as you exhale and engage the core to lower one arm and the opposite leg. You can press a small ball or block onto the thigh if reaching for the leg feels too uncomfortable *(g-h)*.

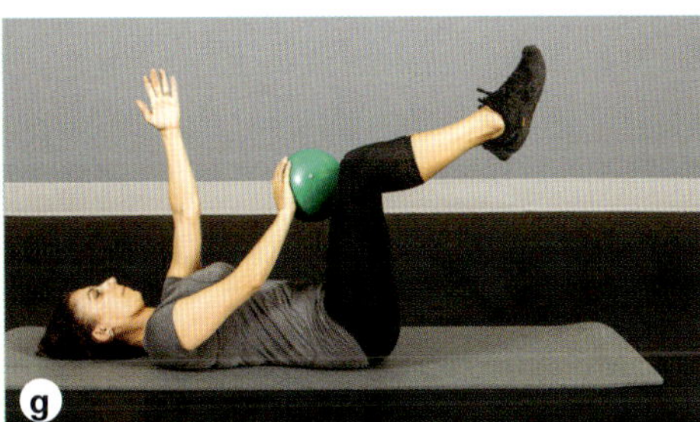
g

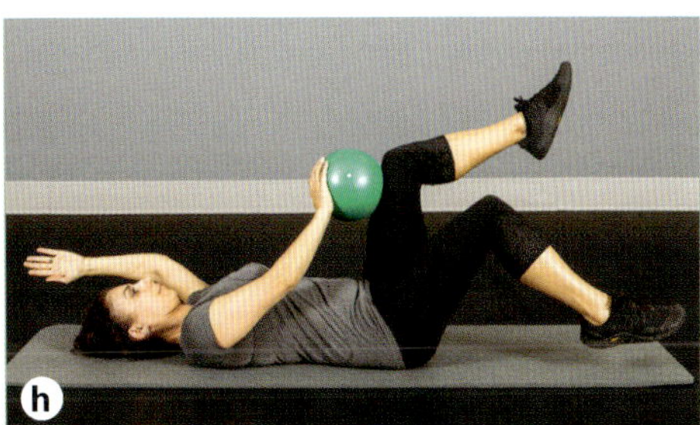
h

Complementary

This secondary list includes more complementary exercises to do if time permits. These exercises will build overall strength, stability, core, and posture and can be performed on alternating days with the foundation exercises. Or you can perform specific exercises based on preference, goals, needs, and time.

WALKING LUNGE WITH BICEPS CURL

The walking lunge is a great exercise that is easily included after a walk. I often do a few sets of walking lunges at the end of a walk or run. Adding the biceps curl allows this exercise to become more compound and integrated. The biceps play a role in helping to maintain that fixed arm angle when walking at higher speeds. The hammer curl (palms facing in) would be a bit more specific to walking; however, the supinated (palms facing up) version is a good option as well. Happy lunging!

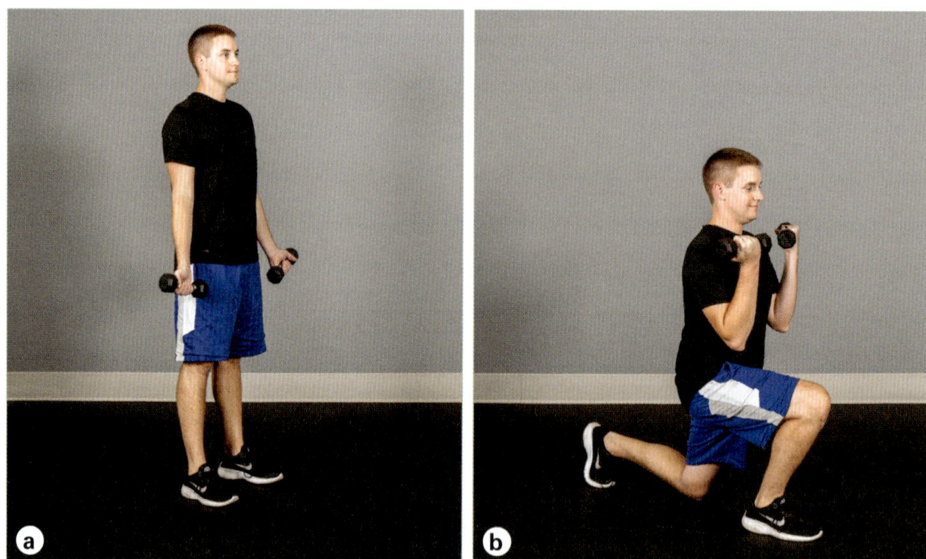

Instructions

Start by standing tall and holding a dumbbell in each hand *(a)*. Take a large step forward and lunge by bending both knees, aiming to create 90-degree angles in each leg *(b)*. Press through the front foot to come up, trying not to push off the back leg. As you come up, perform a biceps curl by bringing both wrists toward the shoulders, palms facing in or up (neutral or supinated grip). As you lower the arms, step forward with the other leg and repeat the lunge and biceps curl. Continue to alternate legs.

Variations

If the walking lunge pattern is challenging, start by stepping back into a reverse lunge pattern. Lunge back to the 90-degree angles and as you press up through the front foot, perform the biceps curl *(c-d)*.

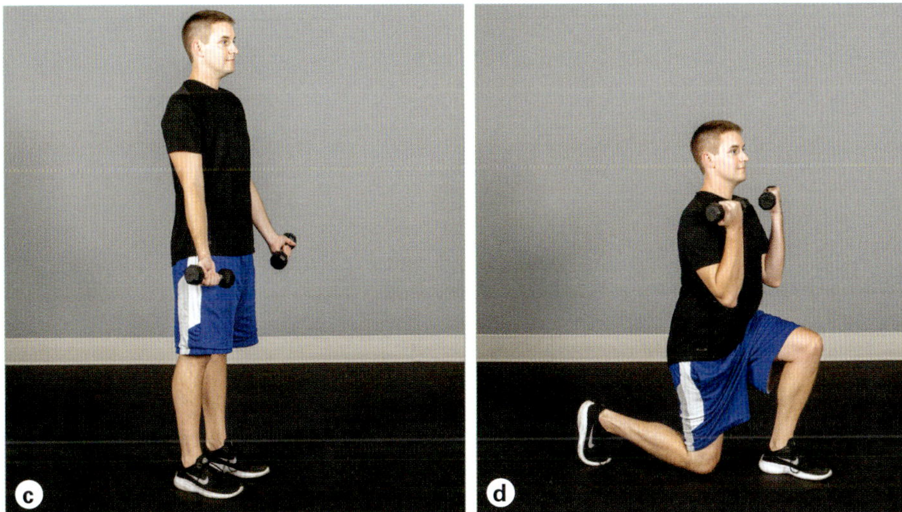

For more of a challenge, increase the weights, slow the tempo, or increase the time of the pause at the top to challenge the balance.

PUSH-UP

The push-up is a convenient, effective, all-in-one exercise that targets the chest, back, triceps, core, shoulders, and more in one movement. It's a "big bang for your buck" exercise that I include in my strength workouts at least once weekly. Many of my clients know that their plans will often include push-ups. It's a love–hate relationship for many! They are effective but challenging!

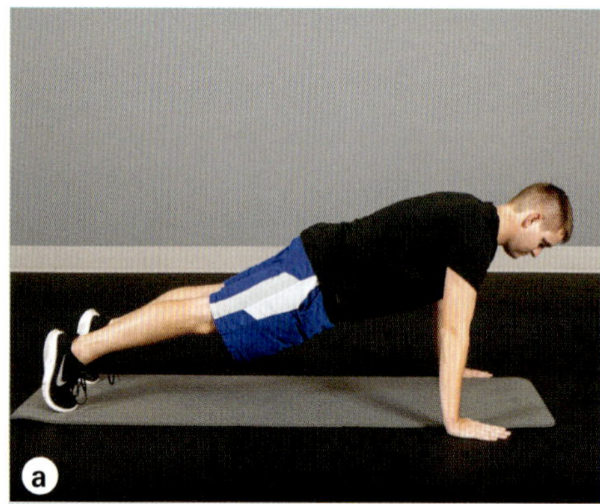
a

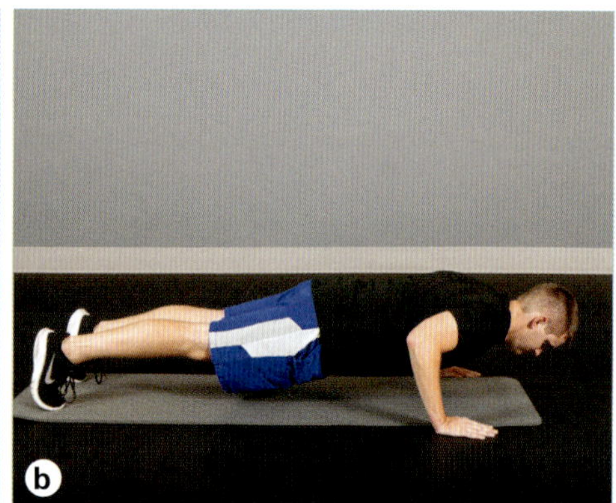
b

Instructions

Start in a high plank position on your hands and feet with your hands in line with your shoulders yet slightly wider than shoulder width and your back in a straight line *(a)*. Push your hands into the floor to prevent sinking in the shoulder blades. Lift your low ribs up to keep your ribs aligned with your hips. Ensure the head, neck, and back are all in alignment. Bend your elbows and lower your chest to the floor, while keeping your body in a straight line *(b)*. Exhale to press up to your start position. Keep your core engaged throughout, though a core break can be taken at the top of the push-up.

Variations

A great starting suggestion is to get comfortable performing the push-ups from your knees. Start with the same hand position but with your knees on the floor *(c)*. Think of placing your body in a straight line from your head to your knees. Lower your chest to the floor while keeping your head in line with your back and your back straight *(d)*. Press back up to your starting point. Push-ups can also be performed on an elevated surface like a counter or bench. Try holding dumbbells if placing your palms flat on the ground is painful.

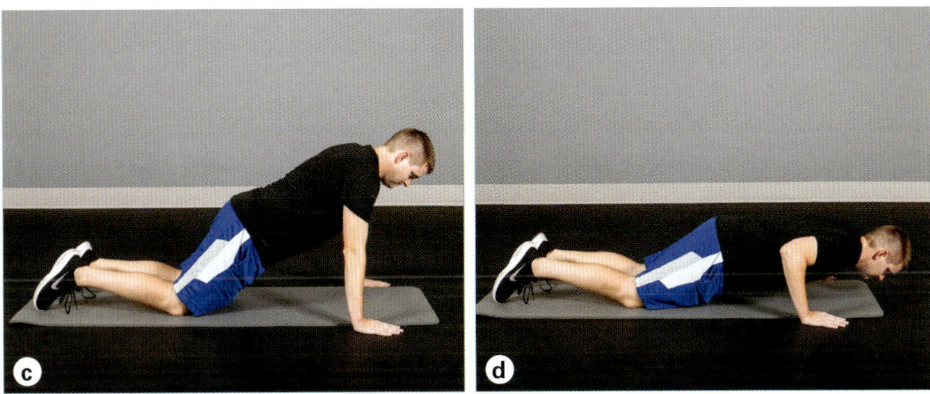

For a greater challenge, perform the push-ups on your toes with one foot elevated *(e-f)*. Perform half the repetitions and switch sides.

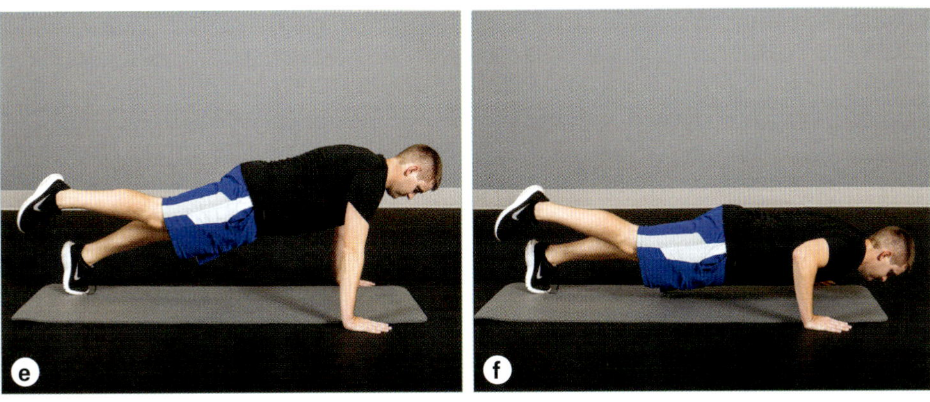

SQUAT JUMPS

Adding some impact work is beneficial to increase bone density. Many of us can include some sort of velocity and power training. Start small and build up slowly to adding more impact and height. Stop if you feel any pain or discomfort. Pay close attention to deceleration or landing mechanics.

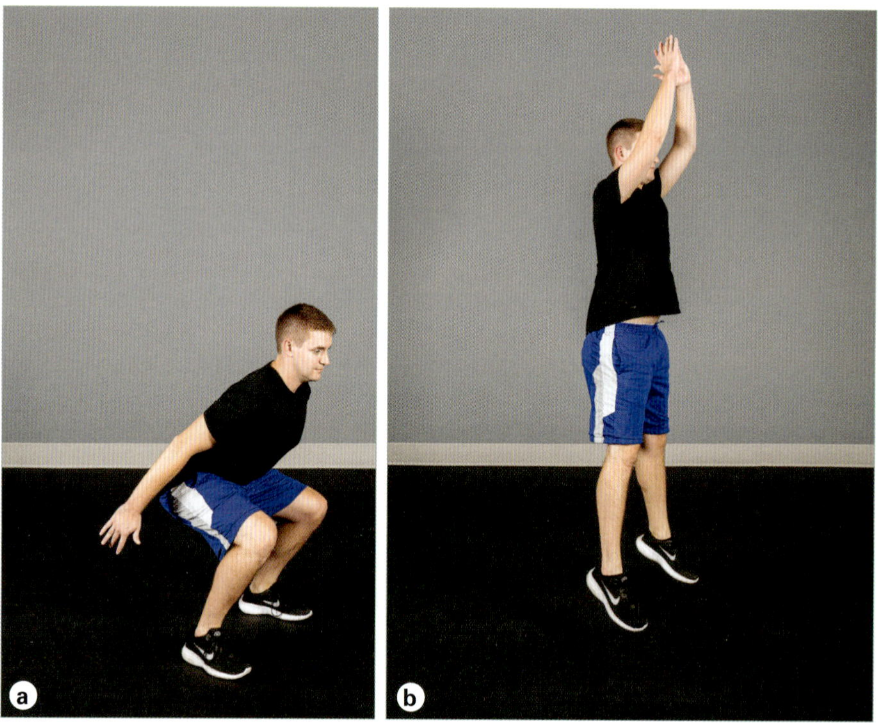

Instructions

Start with your feet shoulder-width apart and your hands by your sides. Squat down and swing your arms behind you, ready for takeoff *(a)*. Drive your hips forward as you jump off the floor, bringing your arms overhead *(b)*. Land softly in a squat position and repeat. Start with small jumps and slowly increase in height and velocity.

Variations

If the thought of jumping is too overwhelming or not possible due to injury, discomfort, or pelvic floor challenges, set up for a squat jump but instead of jumping off the floor, come up onto your toes quickly *(c)*. Sit back down into your squats and repeat, moving fast as you reach up and lift onto the balls of your feet without jumping.

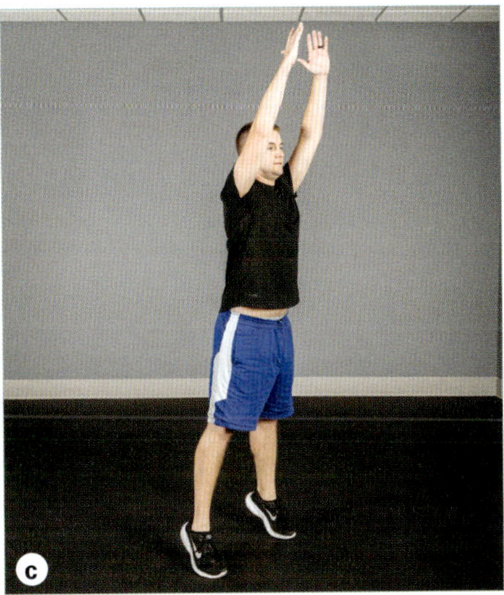

If the squat jump is easy, start the jumps from a split squat position *(d)*. Use both arms to swing up as you jump both feet off the floor at the same time *(e)*. Land with the same leg forward or jump and alternate sides.

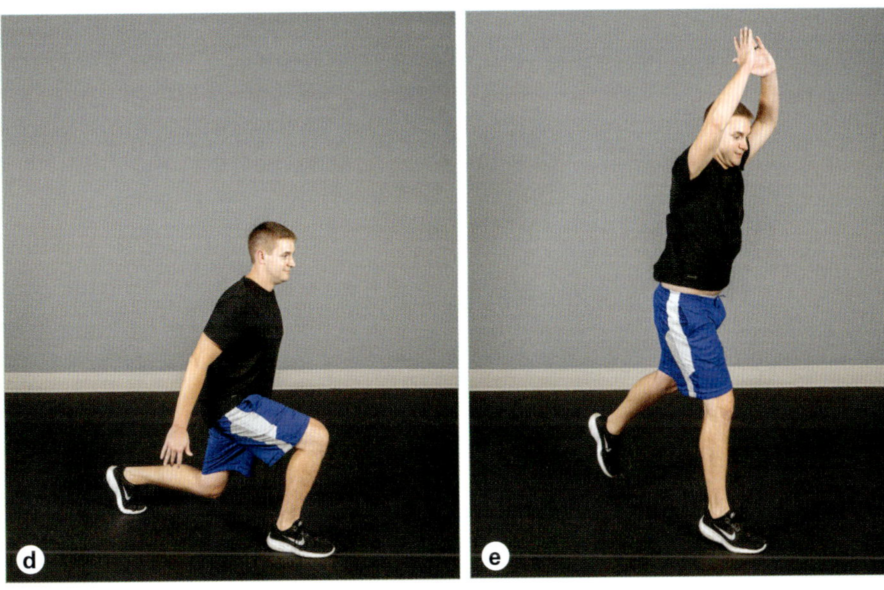

WALL ARM RAISE

As we learned from chapter 4, alignment and posture are important. Our day-to-day activities tend to pull us out of optimal posture. This exercise creates some awareness and focus surrounding our posture and strengthens our postural muscles (back of the shoulders and back area), the muscles that help to keep us tall and well aligned.

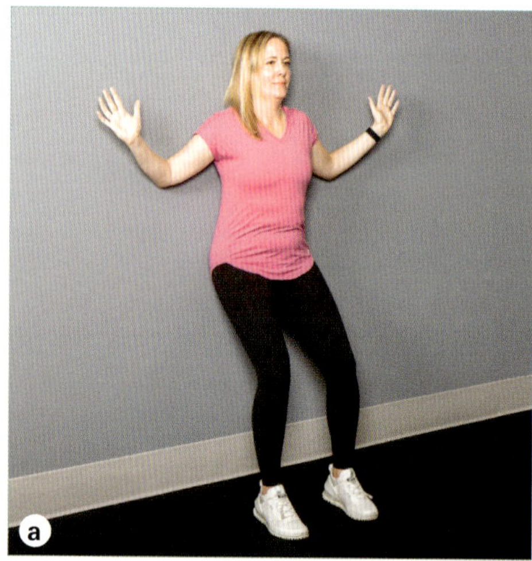
a

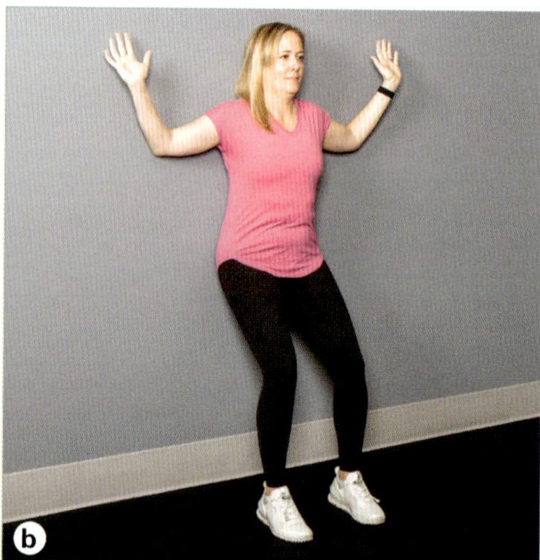
b

Instructions

Start by placing your hips, middle of your back (including low ribs), and your head against a wall. The head may not be able to reach the wall. If not, ensure the chin is parallel to the floor and not jutting upward, to help keep the spine neutral. Bend your knees and place your feet a few inches away from the wall. Place your arms on the wall in a low W position, with your palms facing forward and your elbows close to your rib cage *(a)*. Keep your gaze forward, your chin parallel to the floor, and your shoulders down as you press the back of your hands and arms into the wall. Raise your arms up a couple of inches, maintaining the backward pressure into the wall *(b)*. Lower down to your start position and repeat.

Variations

The wall arm raise can be performed lying down on your back for an easier variation *(c-d)*.

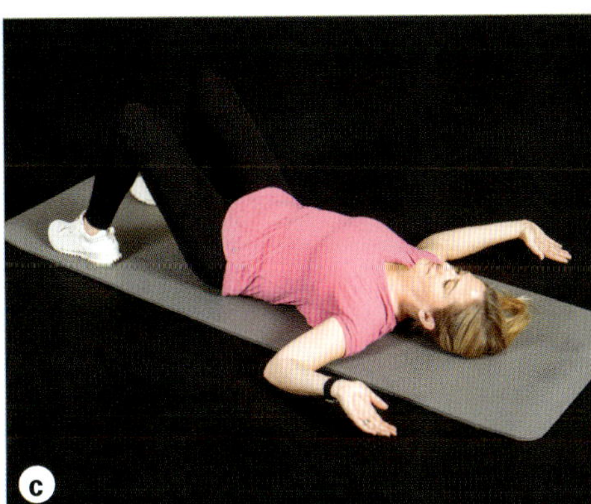
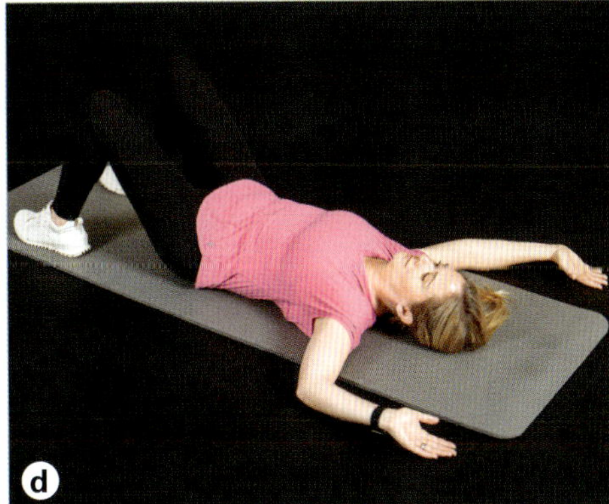

Or try a wall snow angel, which might be better for those experiencing high neck activation. Position the body on the wall as described and place the arms straight back onto the wall about 30 degrees away from the hips *(e)*. Press the arms back into the wall and raise the arms (straight) up a few inches and lower back down *(f)*. For a greater challenge, perform the wall arm raise with greater ranges of motion or greater pressure with the arms pressed back into the wall.

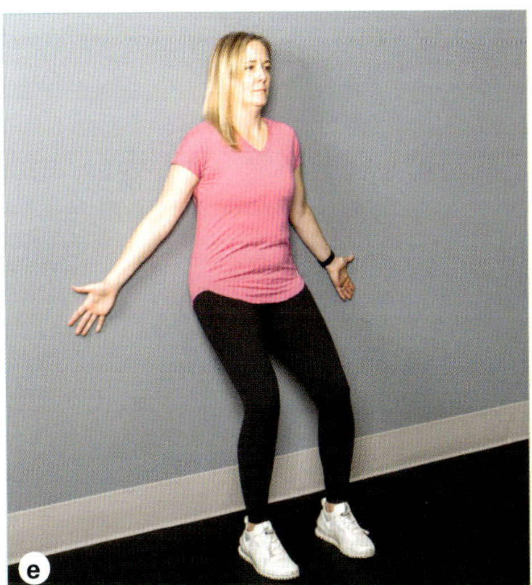
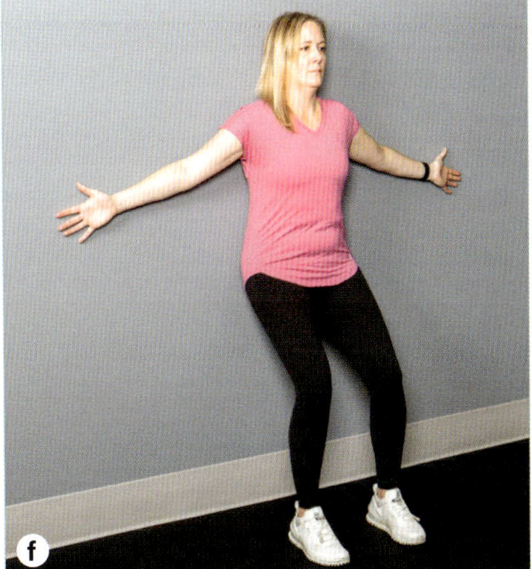

DUMBBELL TRICEPS EXTENSION

Walking involves humeral (arm) extension, and the triceps are a group of muscles that assist this action. This exercise targets the long head of the triceps—that is, the inner line of the triceps or back of the arm. Many of my clients find this area difficult to target and enjoy this particular triceps variation.

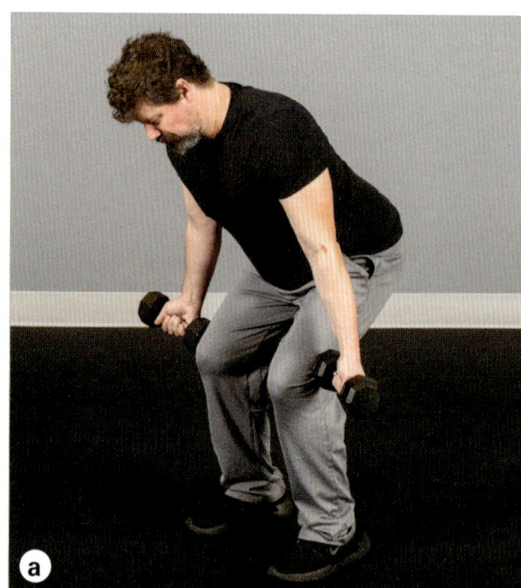
a

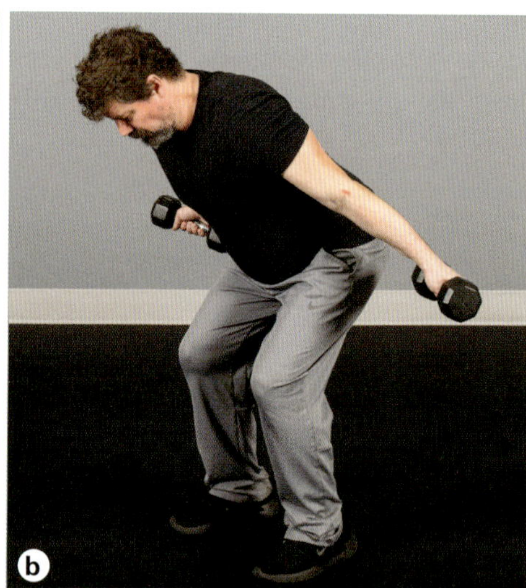
b

Instructions

Hold a dumbbell in each hand and lean forward into a bent-over position with your knees bent and your back flat and straight. Gaze down so that your neck is in line with your spine *(a)*. Keep the arms and the palms facing forward and extend your arms back to the hip line *(b)*. Return to the start position. Continue extending back with the arms straight. The hands will reach the hip line when extended and will return to the knee line once the repetition is complete.

Variations

This exercise can be performed from a seated position if the setup is challenging. Sit at the edge of a chair and move the arms back, ensuring the palms remain facing forward *(c-d)*.

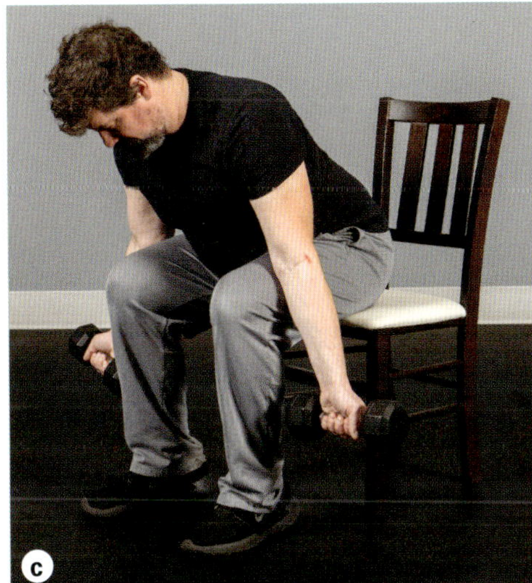

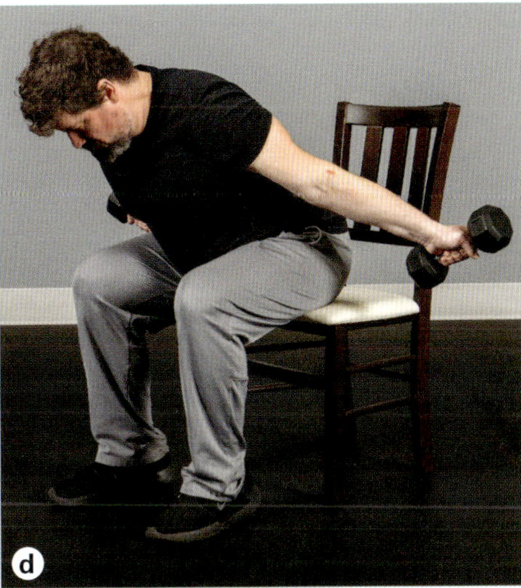

For a more challenging variation, increase the weight, or slow down the tempo.

AXE CHOP

Training rotational patterns is vital to ensure overall balance in the body. Although walking is somewhat linear, including some rotation work will help with our everyday activities. Twisting, rotating, and turning are part of our lives and loading them can help to build our overall fitness.

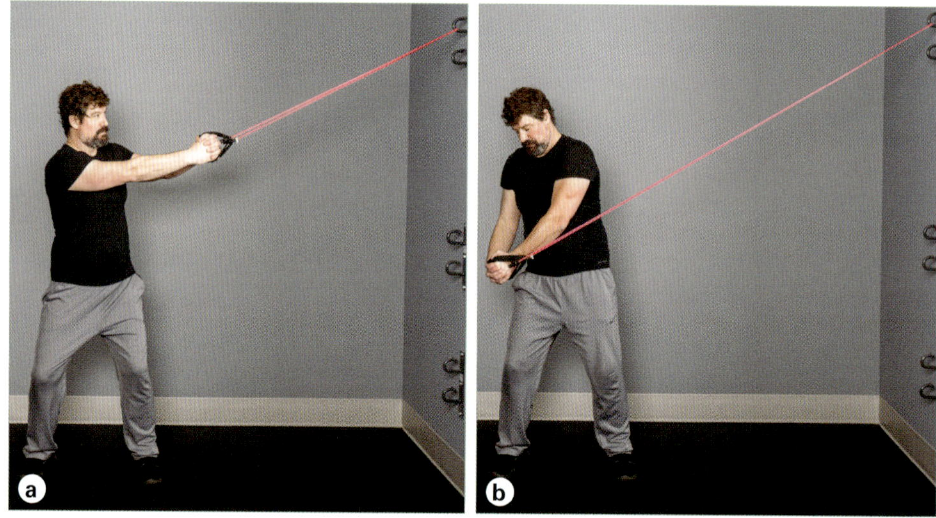

Instructions

Attach a band above shoulder height to a secure object. Stand perpendicular to the band anchor point, with the band in your hands at the inside shoulder level and your feet shoulder-width apart *(a)*. Begin with the hands up at the inside shoulder and slowly pull the band down to the opposite hip, keeping the arms extended *(b)*. Add more tension to the band by standing farther away or using a more difficult band tension. Complete all repetitions, then switch sides.

Variations

If the high-to-low variation is difficult, try performing the axe chop in a low-to-high sequence. Set up the hands holding the band on the inside hip, rotate, and bring the band up to the opposite shoulder, pivoting on the inside foot *(c-d)*.

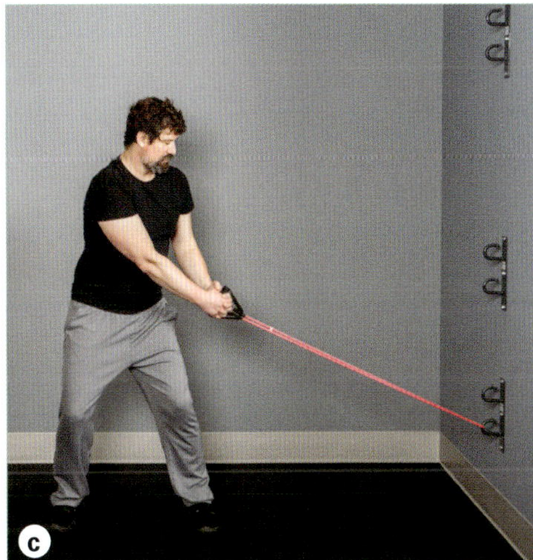

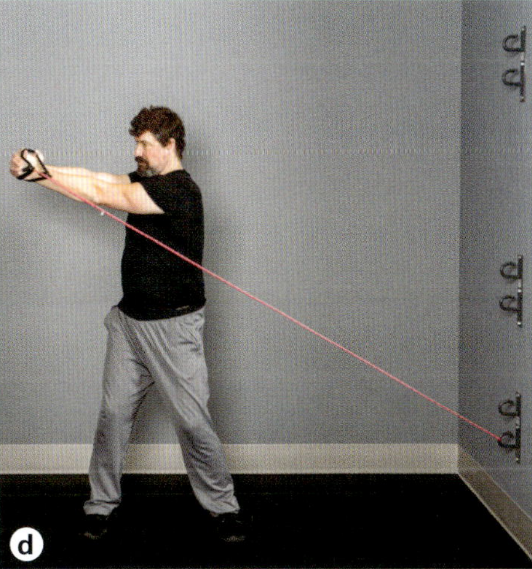

For a greater challenge, stand farther away from your anchor point or use a heavier band resistance. If you have access to a cable system, the axe chop can be performed on the adjustable cable machine, found at many gyms, for a greater challenge. The load can be increased progressively.

SHORT FOOT

Short foot is an excellent exercise that focuses on the intrinsic muscles of the feet. The feet are our literal foundation. When we wear supportive footwear throughout our entire day, we may lose the ability to connect and challenge the deeper muscles in the foot that help to support our arches—and our bodies. Dr. Emily Splichal, functional podiatrist and CEO and founder of Naboso, shares, "Short foot is my go-to foot exercise for strengthening the arch of the foot and for establishing foot-to-core stability. There is an integrated fascial line (deep front line) that runs from the tips of the toes, up the lower leg, through the pelvic floor, and into the diaphragm. When performing short foot, there is an activation of this fascial line and a postural awakening that occurs between our feet, core, and diaphragm. Because of this powerful integration, I use short foot as a way to prep the body for movement." Spending small amounts of time barefoot and including this specific exercise help to increase our overall stability.

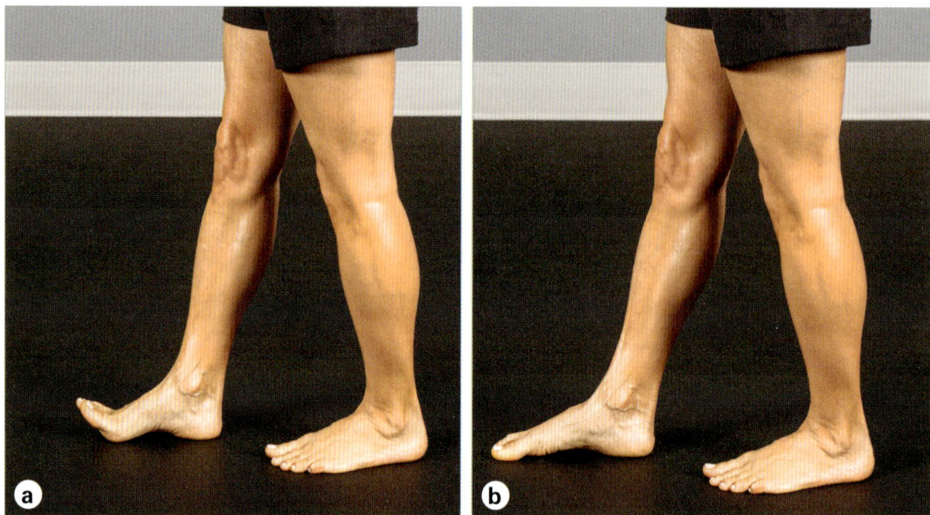

Instructions

Begin by standing with your feet shoulder-width apart. Focus on one foot at a time for this exercise. Lift your toes off the floor, spread your toes wide, and place them down onto the floor *(a)*. Notice when you lift your toes up, you naturally lift your arch off the floor. Maintain this arch lift and press the tips of the toes down into the floor (think of the nail beds pressing down into the floor). At the same time, focus on lifting the arch up, doming the foot, and shortening the foot by trying to bring the toes to the heels *(b)*. Hold this contraction for a few seconds, relax the foot, repeat, then switch to the other foot.

Variations

Hold on to a wall or chair for an easier variation and for more support.

For a greater challenge, shift your weight onto one leg, biasing one foot, and perform the short foot exercise on the stance leg *(c-d)*. Work toward performing short foot on one leg (balancing on one leg). Over time, work to integrate short foot into your strength exercises (e.g., squats, lunges).

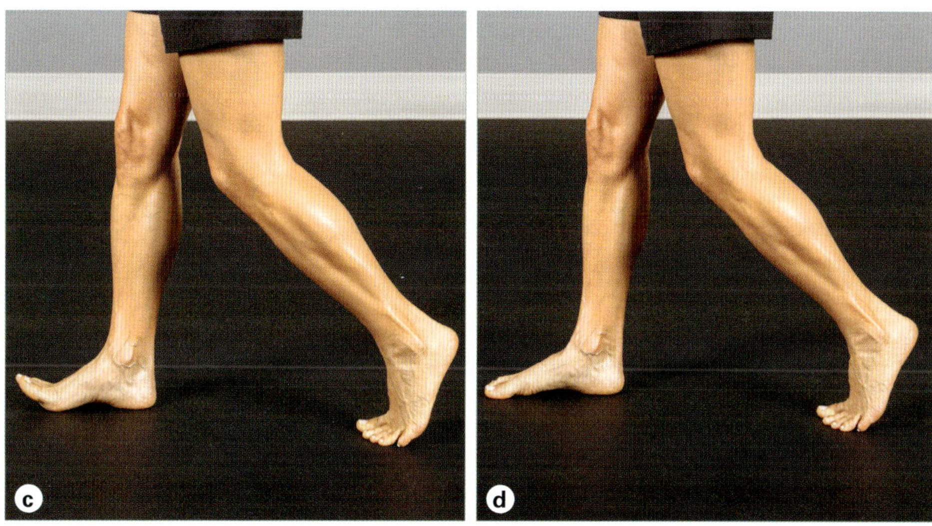

PLANK

Planking can be done in a variety of ways with very different focuses, depending on technique. When planking, try not to clasp your hands together as this shifts load to the chest and shoulders. When up in your plank, focus on the traction element by pulling your ribs to your hips, like a mini crunch. These two changes in the plank can make a big difference, and many of my clients are very surprised when adding these specific cues. Clients who often feel their low backs in a plank may now feel the core and start shaking after only a few seconds.

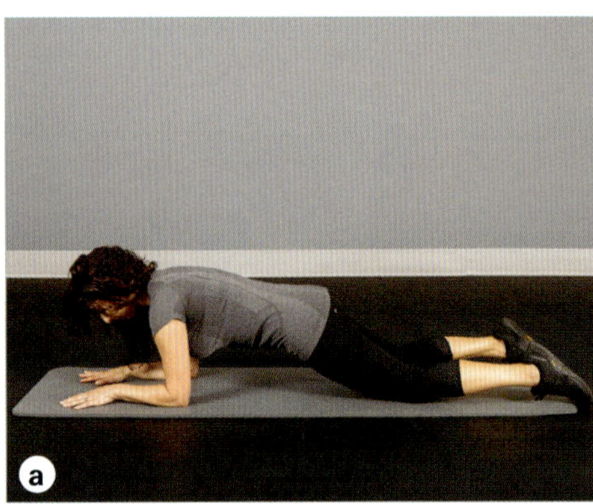
a

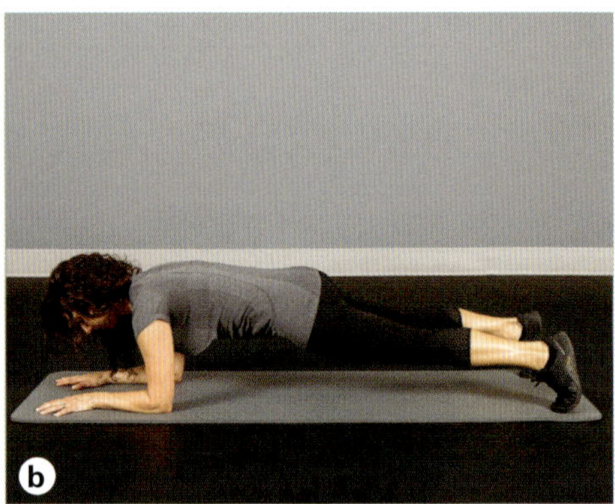
b

Instructions

Lie on your stomach and prop yourself up onto your elbows with your elbows directly under your shoulders. Align your wrists, elbows, and knees *(a)* or toes *(b)* as if they are on train tracks. Slowly lift your ribs, belly, and hips with your knees on the floor until your body forms a straight line. Ensure the low back isn't sinking down to the floor. Lift the low ribs up to smooth out the low back line and look at the floor to keep your head, neck, and back in line. From there, imagine gently pulling your elbows to your knees (without moving the elbows—it's a static pull) and focus on pulling your ribs to your hips like a mini crunch. Hold for as long as possible without feeling any low back tension. Aim for multiple sets of 30-, 45-, or 60-second holds.

Variations

If staying in the plank position on the knees is challenging, try lifting up into the plank position, holding for 5 to 10 seconds, lowering down to take a break, and repeating. Breaking it into smaller chunks will slowly build tolerance.

Some may be more comfortable planking on the hands instead of the elbows or on an elevated surface like a counter or bench *(c)*.

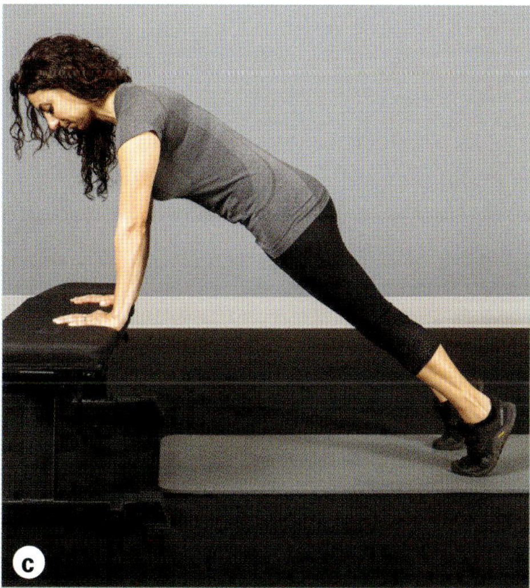

You can hold for longer periods of time to increase the difficulty or lift one leg up and plank on one leg and alternate sides (spend an equal amount of time planking on each leg) *(d)*.

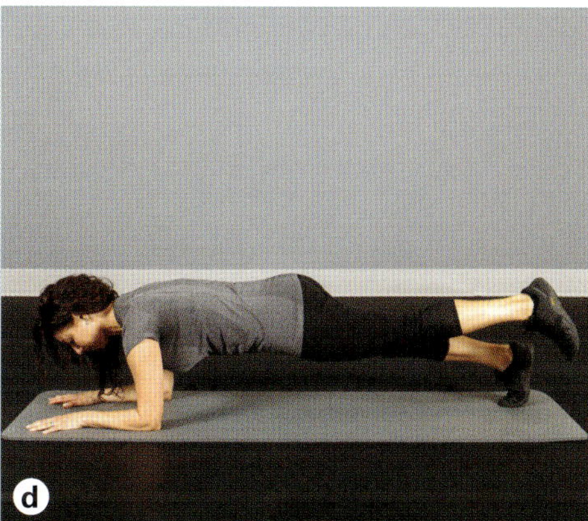

Core Gripping and Glute Gripping

Should I clench my core and glutes when walking? I get asked this question a *lot*! Some clients have been told that one or the other area is weak, so they think about their core or glutes when walking.

Gripping or clenching muscles constantly when walking is not recommended. It's difficult to think about engaging a muscle for 5,000 or 10,000 steps. Muscles need to relax and contract to function optimally. Think of a biceps curl: If you held your arm at the top position all day, your arm and shoulder would fatigue quickly. Try to perform a biceps curl with the arm stuck at the top position, and it just won't fire well. Muscles need to lengthen and extend before contracting fully. The same thing needs to happen with our core and glute muscles. Depending on where we are in the gait cycle, muscles will lengthen and contract as needed. If there is a muscle imbalance, dysfunction, or lack of strength, training them in a controlled environment will provide that functional crossover to walking. Working on proper activations, integrations, loading, and strengthening improves our overall muscle function. That work on our own time will help our muscles respond best when walking, without the need for constant gripping. The work you do at the gym or at home during your strength sessions will train your body and brain to do what is needed to support you.

Another note of caution with gripping regards pressure and joint position. Core gripping (also referred to as *hourglass syndrome*) will affect our intra-abdominal pressure systems, possibly in a negative way. Imagine our abdominal cavity is similar to a balloon. How we breathe, contract our muscles, move, and stand will affect the pressure of this balloon. Constantly gripping our core is similar to squeezing the balloon. The balloon doesn't have an opportunity to expand, and we end up placing excessive intra-abdominal pressure on our backs, pelvic floors, or abdominal walls. This excess pressure may lead to pain, pelvic floor dysfunction, and other potential issues. Jill Miller, C-IAYT, ERYT, author of *Body By Breath* and *The Roll Model* shares,

> Chronic core gripping will limit the diaphragm's ability to plunge downward upon tissues below the ribs during a breath cycle. This downward motion of the diaphragm is necessary for optimal respiratory function. If the abs are held tight, whether consciously or unconsciously, the body will find a workaround for its breath. The body will then develop a new baseline breath that hovers in the rib cage and shoulders. Chronic breathing in the upper trunk is associated with anxiety and negative affect. A body that gets stuck in exclusive chest breathing will also develop stiffness in the muscles of the head, neck, upper back, and shoulders as a result of overusing muscles that should only occasionally be used for breathing. This can lead to pain and other aggravating symptoms in these same areas.

When the core is in a constant state of bracing, this can also inhibit ease of digestion, bowel movements, and challenges with pelvic floor, including sexual pain and urinary or fecal incontinence.

Excessive gripping of our glutes may cause the head of our femur (thigh bone) to be pushed forward in the acetabulum (hip socket). In my personal experience, I've found that many of my clients with hip discomfort, including labral tears, are glute grippers. For some, simply ungripping the glutes can provide relief of symptoms for those with hip pain.

Many of us have been told to always tighten our core (or glutes or other muscles). We may have been taught the notion that we have to pull in our tummies to appear thinner, slimmer, or taller. This constant pulling in is not healthy for our backs, cores, hips, and pelvic floors. Our muscles will contract when needed and, if not, we can train them separately, not by gripping them all day long. Dr. Kathy Dooley, anatomist, chiropractor, creator of Immaculate Dissection, and professor shares, "Waking is dynamic. To grip the core and glutes would compromise the dynamism needed to transition through the phases of gait." Muscles need a break, and our brains need to be rewired to not rely on faulty patterns.

I personally aim to strength train three times per week, focusing on major muscle groups, cleaning up patterns, and lifting heavy most of the time. I include a posture emphasis, core challenge, and more emphasis on the posterior chain (e.g., rear shoulders, back, glutes, hamstrings) to help include more balance in the body. My primary goal is muscle gain and maintenance (as well as overall bone health). Complement your walking with strength training, and your body will thank you!

Now that we've built a solid foundation with form, technique, and alignment and learned the importance of strength training, it's time to put it all into practice. The next few chapters will include numerous walking workouts providing options for varying goals and fitness levels. Whether you have 10, 20, or 30 minutes, there's a time-based workout for you. Turn to the next chapter and dive in!

PART IV

WALKING WORKOUTS AND TRAINING PLANS

CHAPTER 10

Time-Based Workouts

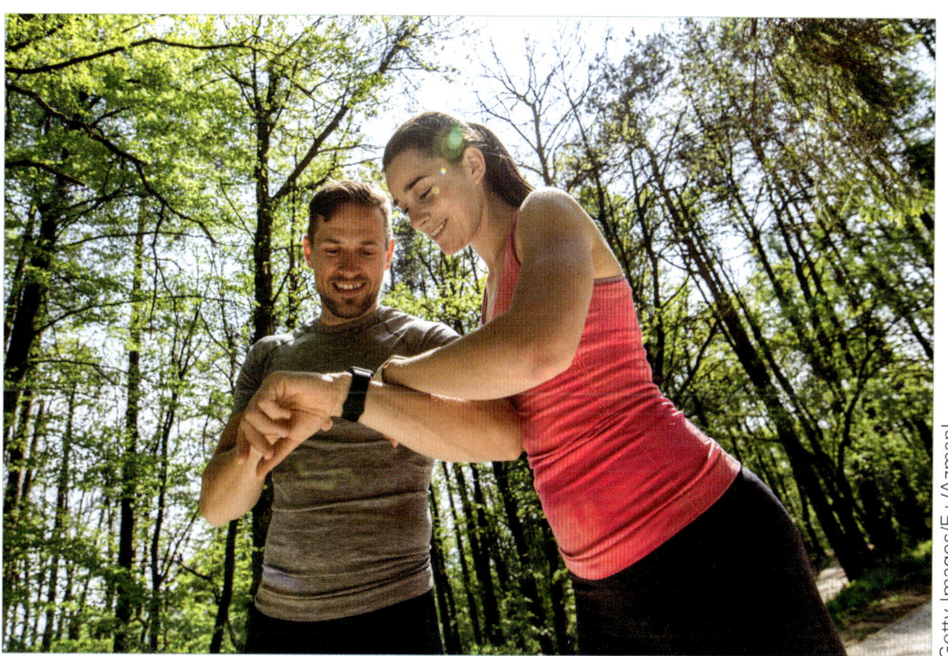

Getty Images/E+/AzmanL

When embarking on a new exercise routine, it's important to start small, progress slowly, pay attention to how we're feeling, and establish clear baselines. Start with 5 to 15 minutes of easy walking as a foundation if you're new to physical activity. At the beginning, aim to be consistent with small amounts. The volumes, intensities, time, and variation will come; first establish a consistent walking routine. The 5- to 15-minute walk is accessible for many, doable, easy to accomplish, and takes less motivation than a longer walk. It can be as simple as parking a few minutes farther away from work to help us easily accumulate walking time or starting with a walk around the block. These regular walks will soon become part of our regular day-to-day activities and eventually we'll think less about it. The more we can automate physical activity, the less bandwidth it takes up in our overall daily routines. We don't think about it—we just go for a walk. Automating our routines allows us to work around what's important, and movement is a big part of what keeps us healthy.

Once you've established your consistent 5- to 15-minute, regular walks, start to progress slowly. In general, aim to add about 10 percent of walking volume each week. Notice how you feel with the added time. If you're feeling pain or discomfort, you can move back to your baseline and aim to increase again from there. Try to ensure moderate to vigorous effort on most days, allowing for occasional slower-paced, lower-intensity, and easier days when you need them. It's okay to periodize and undulate your training. Deloading, lower-intensity, and lower-volume days should all be built into training plans to allow for greater overall recovery.

Various time-based walking workouts are detailed in this chapter. The first level is for those starting out or for experienced walkers needing slightly lower effort on a particular day. The second level provides options for when we're feeling greater levels of energy and strength and can include a bit more volume, speed, and intensity once we've built up a good base.

20-Minute Walk

Studies have shown that walking even short distances can help improve overall health. A 2011 study of 1,000 participants found that those who walked 20 minutes, 5 days per week experienced 43 percent fewer sick days compared to those who were sedentary (Nieman et al. 2011). The quick, 20-minute walk can be a great opportunity to fit in a walk in the morning before work, on your break or lunch hour, or after dinner to help reduce blood sugar increases (table 10.1). Walking after a meal is a great way to help manage overall blood sugar levels and prevent post-meal spikes (Nygaard et al. 2009). Twenty minutes can be an easier target for many to start with. This workout would be a great starting point for those new to exercise, those with hectic schedules, or those looking to slowly increase their activity after a period of being sedentary. The 20-minute walk can also be performed twice daily if schedules don't allow for longer walks. Breaking up walking workouts can be equally effective at improving overall health and wellness. Depending on their ages, the

TABLE 10.1 20-Minute Walking Workout

	Level 1	Level 2
Warm-up	3-5 min	3-5 min
Progressive build to walking pace	3-5 min	1-3 min
Walking speed/time	Moderate: 10 min	Moderate to fast: 15 min
Interval break	1 min	N/A
Cool-down	5 min	2-5 min
Stretch (optional)	5 min	5 min

postmeal, 20-minute walk is a great option for the whole family to enjoy some physical activity while spending time together.

30-Minute Walk

According to experts, North Americans as well as many other populations should be obtaining 150 minutes of moderate- to vigorous-intensity aerobic exercise per week as well as muscle-strengthening activities two or three times per week for overall health (U.S. Department of Health and Human Services 2018; Canadian Society for Exercise Physiology 2021). Older adults should incorporate balance training into their overall fitness plan. The 150 minutes of aerobic activity can be broken down in different ways. Thirty minutes 5 days a week will meet those targets. The guidelines are established to help our populations prevent disease and work toward optimal health. Although this book primarily discusses walking, I recommend varying activities for overall health and wellness whenever possible. Performing different aerobic activities allows our bodies to build tolerance and increase overall thresholds to handle our daily demands. If most of your cardiovascular activity is dedicated to walking, aim to add an additional varied activity once every week or two to provide diversity and variability to your daily movements.

The 30-minute walk is perfect to ensure we're getting our recommended physical activity levels (table 10.2). It's long enough to give us that feeling of having done something (especially if we're pushing it), yet short enough to squeeze into a lunch break without taking too much time away from the workday or other daily activities. Warm up and cool down to ease in and out of your desired pace. When time allows, including some static stretches for the quads, hamstrings, glutes, shins, back, and calves is a great way to round off your walk (see chapter 6 for detailed dynamic warm-up drills, cool-down suggestions, and static stretches).

TABLE 10.2 30-Minute Walking Workout

	Level 1	Level 2
Warm-up	3-5 min	3-5 min
Progressive build to walking pace	5 min	1-3 min
Walking time	15-20 min	20-25 min
Walking pace	Moderate	Moderate to fast
Interval breaks	1 min after every 10 min	1 min after 15 min if needed
Cool-down	5 min	2-5 min
Stretch (optional)	5 min	5 min

45-Minute Walk

The 45-minute walk is a great choice if you want to add more volume, build endurance, increase workout difficulty, and add technical challenges such as intervals and varied terrain (table 10.3). It's longer than the quick 30-minute walk but not as time consuming as a 60-minute walk. This workout is a great choice if you find the 30-minute walks easy but find the 60-minute walk daunting or overwhelming. When selecting this workout, ensure you've done several speedy 30-minute walks first. Take a bit of time progressing to the 45-minute walk. If you increase volume by 10 percent each week, it would in theory take 5 to 6 weeks of slow buildup, allowing plenty of time for the body to adapt to the increased time on your feet. Of course, if you are an athletic individual accustomed to long walks and time on your feet, the ramp-up may be quicker. See how your body feels as you add on the extra mileage and adjust as needed. Some may need extra time to progress, added stretches, longer cool-downs, and extra recovery time between walks if the body needs a reset. Take the time to warm up with some of the dynamic walking drills outlined in chapter 6; many of the warm-up drills can be performed as you're walking and easing into your desired pace.

TABLE 10.3 45-Minute Walking Workout

	Level 1	Level 2
Warm-up	3-5 min	3-5 min
Progressive build to walking pace	5 min	1-3 min
Walking time	30 min	30-35 min
Walking pace	Moderate	Moderate to fast
Interval breaks	1 min after every 10 min	1 min after 15 min if needed
Cool-down	5 min	2-5 min
Stretch (optional)	5 min	5 min

60-Minute Walk

The 60-minute walk is a great option for those who want to add longer walks on weekends, days off, holidays, or those who want to build endurance for 10Ks, half-marathon races, or vacations filled with long sightseeing or beach walks (table 10.4). Many will fill their weekdays with shorter 30-minute walks, leaving weekends for opportunities to walk longer. As we increase time on our feet, good movement preparation becomes more important. In the past, I would often head out the

TABLE 10.4 60-Minute Walking Workout

	Level 1	Level 2
Warm-up	3-5 min	3-5 min
Progressive build to walking pace	5 min	1-3 min
Walking time	45 min	45-50 min
Walking pace	Moderate	Moderate to fast
Interval breaks	1 min after every 10 min	1 min after 15 min if needed
Cool-down	5 min	2-5 min
Stretch (optional)	5 min	5 min

door for outdoor activities, skipping warm-ups, movement preparations, and dynamic stretches, and immediately regretting it as the impacts felt more noted in my body. I've learned to spend a few short minutes with some dynamic preparations, to actively stretch, and to ease into desired walking paces (or with any other physical activity), which feels much better from a muscle, joint, and overall body perspective. Take time to prepare for the longer walks so that the beginnings and ends of the higher volumes may feel better, stronger, and more comfortable. You may find with proper movement preparation that you have the capacity to walk for longer periods with more comfort.

75-Minute Walk

Although not for the fainthearted, the 75-minute walks allow you to build up endurance, walking capacity, and grit (table 10.5). They may be helpful in preparing for trips with longer sightseeing walks, hiking trips, or for days when you know you will be on your feet for long periods of time. Ensure you have several 60-minute walks under your belt

TABLE 10.5 75-Minute Walking Workout

	Level 1	Level 2
Warm-up	3-5 min	3-5 min
Progressive build to walking pace	5 min	1-3 min
Walking time	50-55 min	60-70 min
Walking pace	Moderate	Moderate to fast
Interval breaks	1 min after every 10 min	1 min after 15 min if needed
Cool-down	5 min	2-5 min
Stretch (optional)	5 min	5 min

before embarking on the longer 75-minute walk. Pay attention to your feet, ankles, knees, hips, and back. Are you noticing certain symptoms begin with a specific walking distance or intensity? For example, you notice that you can walk comfortably at a good walking pace but once you walk beyond 60 minutes, you start to experience discomfort such as pain in your heels, shins, or hips. If that is the case, keep your walks just below this threshold (55 minutes in this example) and work to incorporate strength elements to help build tissue tolerance. Seeing a physiotherapist or other health care professional can help treat the issue. You may need to modify rather than stop the activity altogether. After a few weeks of specific and purposeful strengthening, try to increase your walking time slowly (10% volume each week) and see if you're now able to walk a bit longer before the symptoms creep up. If your baseline is now 65 minutes, then follow this same strategy (walk 60 minutes and continue to strengthen, etc.). This progressive strategy can keep you moving, address underlying issues, and build your thresholds for higher volumes without experiencing discomfort.

Time Trial

The time trial is a great opportunity to assess walking fitness at any point in time (table 10.6). It can be any length of time you choose. If you tend to walk speedy for short distances, aim for a 5- or 10-minute time trial. If you enjoy longer walks, try a 20-minute time trial to establish baselines and measure progress.

Start your timer and walk as fast as you comfortably can for the desired time. Plan to reassess at regular intervals. Bimonthly or a few times annually would be reasonable intervals to measure progress. More frequent assessment would likely not show results of regular training. Ideally, reassess at similar intervals using the same conditions: same route, same terrain (e.g., sidewalk, track, trail), same time of day, fasted or not fasted, and so on. For women, assess at the same time of month because energy tends to fluctuate with individual infradian rhythms.

TABLE 10.6 Time Trial

	5 min time trial	10 min time trial	20 min time trial
Warm-up	3-5 min	3-5 min	3-5 min
Time trial	5 min	10 min	20 min
Cool-down	3-5 min	3-5 min	3-5 min
Stretch	5 min	5 min	5 min

These walking workouts are suggestions for those who want to add some structure and challenge to their overall routine. Take the time to warm up and cool down properly and add static stretches at the end of the walk to improve overall range of motion and comfort. If a walking workout feels difficult or challenging, try the lower-level option or the shorter option and slowly work your way up to your desired time-based workout. Ensure you've performed a number of these steady-state walking workouts before attempting more technical, purpose-based workouts (chapter 11). If you experience pain that lingers after your walk, see a health professional to treat the issue early on. Addressing an injury at the first sign of symptoms saves much time (and pain) later on.

CHAPTER 11

Purpose-Based Workouts

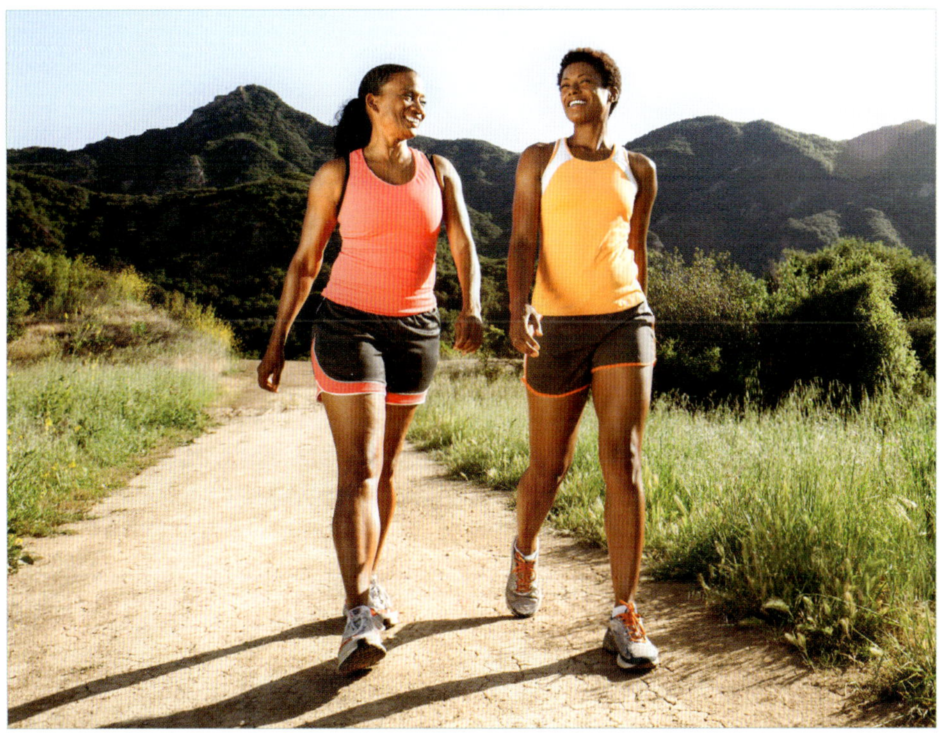

Erik Isakson/Tetra images RF/Getty Images

You've established some consistent, steady-state walks and are ready for more. Or you're ready for more variety and more of a challenge with your walks. Maybe you're someone who wants to get the most out of your walks. This is the chapter for you. Many don't really consider walking as physical activity or feel it counts. With these walking workouts, it counts! You'll be able to elevate your heart rate, recruit different muscles, recruit muscles in a fuller capacity, increase cardiac output, build cardiovascular endurance, and boost the overall challenge of your walks. They have been curated for the beginner, intermediate, and advanced walker and there arc various options to choose from.

Hills

Walking (or running) uphill is easily one of my favorite activities to include in my programming. It's effective, challenging, easier on the joints, and increases the heart rate. In one study, researchers found that walking uphill significantly increases heart rate versus walking on level surfaces or downhill (Adhikari and Patil 2018). Another study found that incline walking decreases impacts on the leg and provides muscle-strengthening effects (Masood and Kobsar 2021). Women who experience pelvic floor challenges may find walking uphill an effective alternative to higher-impact activities.

We've outlined some suggested hill workouts in table 11.1. If you live in a fairly flat area, climbing stairs can be an alternative. Driving to a hillier location if that's possible might be another option. If you only have one very large hill available, you can start by walking part way up the hill (for the allotted time) and increase the time or distance as you become more comfortable.

If walking downhill is challenging, scout out routes ahead of time that will allow you to walk uphill and perhaps level out a bit on streets or trails to ease stress off the knees. Descending recruits much more of the quadriceps muscles in an eccentric fashion. Climbing up stairs in a building and taking the elevator down can be an option to offload the knees. Walking up a flight or two of stairs and walking down the hall will break up the climbs and descents. If those options aren't realistic for you, find different ways to descend, such as side stepping for short periods of time, which may be more comfortable. Warm up prior to the hill workout and cool down and stretch afterward.

TABLE 11.1 Hill Walking Workout

	Level 1	Level 2	Level 3	Level 4
Warm-up	3-5 minutes	3-5 minutes	3-5 minutes	3-5 minutes
Hill distance	20-30 second climb	35-45 second climb	50-60 second climb	30 seconds
Hill repeats	1-3	4-5	6-8	2-3
Active walking break between hills	2-3 minutes	1-2 minutes	45-60 seconds	2-3 min
Walking speed	Slow to moderate	Moderate	Moderate to fast	Max effort
Cool-down	5 minutes	5 minutes	5 minutes	5 minutes
Stretch (optional)	5 minutes	5 minutes	5 minutes	5 minutes

Interval Training

Interval training is not a new form of activity. Exercisers have been performing variations of interval training for years. Our ancestors have been performing this type of movement modality for centuries. It's characterized by performing short bursts of intense activity followed by a period of rest or low-intensity exercise. It's functional, purposeful, effective, and challenging. It adds variety to workouts and gives an added boost of physiological adaptations. Research has shown that high-intensity interval training improves exercise capacity, including maximal oxygen uptake, aerobic endurance, and anaerobic capacity as well as improved metabolic health (in active and inactive individuals) (Atakan et al. 2021).

In the following suggested workouts, we've included options for interval training (table 11.2). We're aiming to work as hard as possible when pushing through an interval, following up with slower periods of walking to actively recover between interval sets. The longer periods of intervals in level 3 are meant to work on improving $\dot{V}O_2$max capacity, which is an outcome measure of our physical fitness. Our $\dot{V}O_2$max measures the maximum amount of oxygen our bodies use while exercising. In the longer intervals in level 3, the effort will be slightly less intense than our full out, shorter intervals.

Before pushing in the high-intensity zones, ensure you've had several weeks of consistent walking and training under your belt. Warm up actively and dynamically and cool down after each interval workout. These specific workouts might warrant stretching afterward to help feel more comfort after the workout. Proper walking form and technique are required for all levels of intensity. Form may be one determining factor of our upper thresholds of intensity. You should only go as hard as your form can be maintained.

TABLE 11.2 Interval Walking Workout

	Level 1	Level 2	Level 3
Warm-up	3-5 minutes	3-5 minutes	3-5 minutes
Interval distance	30 seconds	45-60 seconds	90 seconds to 4 minutes
Interval repeats	3-5	6-8	2-5
Active walking break between intervals	2-5 minutes	1-2 minutes	1-2 minutes
Walking speed	Slow to moderate	Moderate	Moderate to fast
Cool-down	5 minutes	5 minutes	5 minutes
Stretch (optional)	5 minutes	5 minutes	5 minutes

Power Walk

Many of you may focus your efforts on the power walk. It's nothing fancy—no added skills, drills, bells, or whistles. Just a speedy walk out in your neighborhood or with friends on your favorite routes. These are the walks that we perform time and time again: our go-to walk. My definition of a power walk is walking at a pace that is slightly faster than your comfortable walking pace while maintaining good form and alignment. You'll want to warm up and maintain a quick pace for the length of your walk, keeping in mind all the technical elements we covered in previous chapters. Walking breaks are built in if needed but if you'd rather omit them, that's okay too. There are options for shorter and longer walks. Select the one that fits best into your schedule and works well for you (table 11.3).

TABLE 11.3 Power Walking Workout

	Level 1	Level 2	Level 3
Warm-up	3-5 minutes	3-5 minutes	3-5 minutes
Power walk	20 minutes	30 minutes	45-60 minutes
Walking break	1 minute every 10	1 minute every 15	N/A
Walking speed	Slow to moderate	Moderate	Moderate to fast
Cool-down	5 minutes	5 minutes	5 minutes
Stretch (optional)	5 minutes	5 minutes	5 minutes

Jogging or Running

Many runners walk, and many walkers run. It's not uncommon at running races to see participants running 10 minutes followed by a 1-minute walk. Walking faster during your 1-minute walking break during a running race can help runners finish races faster and avoid losing precious minutes. However, many walkers enjoy being outdoors and on their feet, and they get to a point where they feel jogging or running might be in their realm of possibilities. If this is you, aim to ease into jogging or running slowly, progressively, and intuitively. Table 11.4 provides some suggestions on how to add in short jogging intervals, where each level aims to jog or run more and walk less. Pay attention to what you feel during and after your sessions. Are there any particularly tight or sore areas? A longer warm-up, cool-down, and stretch may be warranted when trying higher-impact activities like jogging or running.

TABLE 11.4 Jog or Run Walking Workout

	Level 1	Level 2	Level 3
Warm-up	3-5 minutes	3-5 minutes	3-5 minutes
Jogging time	30 seconds	45-60 seconds	60-90 seconds
Walking time	90 seconds	60 seconds	30 seconds
Number of jogging intervals	1-3	4-6	8-10
Walking/jogging speed	Slow to moderate	Moderate	Moderate to fast
Cool-down	5 minutes	5 minutes	5 minutes
Stretch (optional)	5 minutes	5 minutes	5 minutes

Treadmill

Walking on a treadmill, as discussed in chapter 3, can be a great option to remain consistent. Whether it's weather challenges (e.g., heat, cold), terrain challenges, uncertain environments, or the need for specificity with time, speed, or distance, the treadmill offers the perfect solution to continue walking. Treadmills often have predetermined programs that many can take advantage of, and I would certainly recommend exploring the options available to you. Some of the preset programs you might find on any commercial or home treadmill include hills, intervals, weight loss or fat burn, heart rate, performance, 5K, and possibly others.

Treadmill workouts provide many options for variety, challenge, and cardiovascular endurance (tables 11.5-11.7).

TABLE 11.5 Treadmill Walking Workout: Hills

	Level 1	Level 2	Level 3
Warm-up	3-5 minutes	3-5 minutes	3-5 minutes
2 minutes	Incline level 3	Incline level 4	Incline level 5
2 minutes	Incline level 4	Incline level 5	Incline level 6
2 minutes	Incline level 5	Incline level 6	Incline level 7
2 minutes	Incline level 6	Incline level 7	Incline level 8
2 minutes	Incline level 5	Incline level 6	Incline level 7
2 minutes	Incline level 4	Incline level 5	Incline level 6
2 minutes	Incline level 3	Incline level 4	Incline level 5
2 minutes	Jump to cool down	Incline level 3	Incline level 4
2 minutes	N/A	Jump to cool down	Incline level 3
Cool-down	5 minutes	5 minutes	5 minutes
Stretch (optional)	5 minutes	5 minutes	5 minutes

TABLE 11.6 Treadmill Walking Workout: Intervals

	Level 1	Level 2	Level 3
Warm-up	3-5 minutes	3-5 minutes	3-5 minutes
Interval 1 Recovery	30 seconds 60 seconds	45-60 seconds 45-60 seconds	60-90 seconds 30-45 seconds
Interval 2 Recovery	30 seconds 60 seconds	45-60 seconds 45-60 seconds	60-90 seconds 30-45 seconds
Interval 3 Recovery	30 seconds 60 seconds	45-60 seconds 45-60 seconds	60-90 seconds 30-45 seconds
Interval 4 Recovery	30 seconds 60 seconds	45-60 seconds 45-60 seconds	60-90 seconds 30-45 seconds
Interval 5 Recovery	30 seconds 60 seconds	45-60 seconds 45-60 seconds	60-90 seconds 30-45 seconds
Interval 6 Recovery	30 seconds 60 seconds	45-60 seconds 45-60 seconds	60-90 seconds 30-45 seconds
Interval 7 Recovery	Jump to cool down N/A	45-60 seconds 45-60 seconds	60-90 seconds 30-45 seconds
Interval 8 Recovery	N/A N/A	Jump to cool down N/A	60-90 seconds 30-45 seconds
Cool-down	5 minutes	5 minutes	5 minutes
Stretch (optional)	5 minutes	5 minutes	5 minutes

TABLE 11.7 Treadmill Walking Workout: Speed

	Level 1	Level 2	Level 3
Warm-up	3-5 minutes	3-5 minutes	3-5 minutes
Pace	Moderate	Moderate to fast	Fast
Walking time	10-15 minutes	15-20 minutes	20-30 minutes
Suggested walking speed	2.5-3 mph (4-5 km/hr)	3.75-4.5 mph (6-7 km/hr)	5+ mph (8+ km/hr)
Cool-down	5 minutes	5 minutes	5 minutes
Stretch (optional)	5 minutes	5 minutes	5 minutes

Trail Walks or Hiking

Trail walks or hikes are a great option for those who love being out in nature, those who live close to the woods or trails with varied terrain, those who enjoy variety when walking, or those who are training for specific hikes, climbs, or destinations that include moderate to significant elevation. I've worked with clients preparing for popular trails such as the Santiago trails in Spain, clients who prepared to climb certain mountains or long hikes with significant elevation, and clients who want to be comfortable hiking with family or friends with the goal being to keep up and feel comfortable on single-day or multiday hikes. In these preparatory sessions, we're aiming to increase strength through specific single-leg strength training, core training, and walking with elevation. We may also walk with weighted packs (rucking) to help prepare the body for the loads hikers will be carrying (e.g., water, food, supplies).

If you're planning a big hike or climb, include some form of hill training or hiking in terrain similar to what you're going to encounter. If you're training to climb a mountain with a 2,000-foot elevation, try to fit in hikes that include some elevation where possible. It may require driving on occasion to fit in these specific training hikes; however, having some specificity in your training will help prepare you for what's to come.

If you're planning a multiday hike or climb, fit in training walks or hikes that are on consecutive days to prepare your body for back-to-back hikes. The work-up to long, multiday hikes takes time and is very individualized. There are many factors that may determine someone's starting point, including level of physical activity, injury, history, weather, and tolerance to heat, humidity, and elevation. Include plenty of time to work up to these hikes or climbs, starting with smaller levels of elevation and gradually work your way up, aiming to increase volume by 10 percent each week.

Winter Walk

Walking in the winter can be a workout all on its own! If you live in a snowy climate, winters can be a challenge. It can be cold, icy, snowy, windy, and difficult to remain consistent with walking. You must be well dressed and well equipped. We discussed important clothing and gear considerations in chapter 3. Once you have the right clothing, increase the challenge when walking in the winter by walking on snowy surfaces, whether hardpacked or not. Snowshoeing is a great option for those looking to continue walking throughout the winter, and it will increase the challenge versus walking on a more stable surface. Snowshoeing, depending on the depth and hardpack nature of the snow, will require more energy and muscle recruitment. You'll likely sink into a snow surface more and you'll need to pick your feet up higher.

The energy expended during snowshoeing will be variable, depending on how hardpacked the snow is, but can require up to 50 percent more energy than walking. Snowshoeing on packed snow at around 3 miles per hour elicited a similar heart rate and energy response to walking on a treadmill at 4 miles per hour or snowshoeing in unpacked snow at 2 miles per hour, according to a study by Connolly (2002). Connolly also showed that snowshoeing on packed snow at around 4 miles per hour elicited the same heart rate and energy expenditure response as walking on a treadmill at 6 miles per hour or snowshoeing on unpacked snow at 3 miles per hour. The study concludes that increasing walking speed on snow by just 1 mph at slow speeds (2 and 3 mph) resulted in approximately twice the energy expenditure. Snowshoeing and walking on packed or unpacked snow provides a greater challenge from an energy and muscle perspective, provides variety with regard to terrain, and helps us to remain consistent during difficult weather challenges.

Dog Walking

We broke down a bit of the mechanics of dog walking in chapter 5 and how it might affect our overall gait. Many dog owners will likely spend the majority of their walks walking their dog. While we don't have any specific dog-walking workouts, varying your walking routes, adding varied terrain such as hills or trails, and picking up the pace in general can add more of a challenge when walking with your dog.

First, if possible, aim to encourage less pulling. This is not easy by any means. We learned the hard way with our first dog. If possible, spend the time early on training loose leash walking or using tools such as harnesses and gentle leaders to encourage less pulling overall. This will help put less strain on your body, encourage better balance and symmetry, and possibly prevent overuse injuries or discomforts.

Next, try to switch the arm holding the leash when walking your dog. Switching sides can help to create balance between right and left sides and prevent overusing one side. We can balance the rotational forces overall by alternating time spent holding the leash in one hand. Another option is to spend some time walking your dog in designated off-leash areas to give your hands, arms, and shoulders a bit of a break.

Finally, plan for frequent stops. Our pups take lots of pauses for smelling, meeting new friends, and taking care of their business. Even though the walk may not be continuous in nature, it still counts as we're on our feet creating forward motion.

Stroller Walk

Although our kids are older now, I have vivid memories of spending hours pushing our children in strollers. John and I knew early on in the pregnancy that we wanted to invest in a durable, versatile, and high-quality stroller. The one we ended up with worked well for walking and running and had attachments for cycling and skiing. Our kids joined us from a young age on all our active adventures. Strollers have changed a great deal over the last 10 to 15 years with more options, selection, and styles. One thing remains: Going out for a walk is great for a baby and great for mom and dad too! It gives new parents an opportunity to get some fresh air and movement, allow the baby to sleep (hopefully!), and brings a fresh perspective to the day.

When walking with the stroller, keep in mind a few key points to remain comfortable. First, stand tall and avoid leaning over at the hips. It can be easy to rest our weight on the handles and bend forward; however, this may place additional strain on the back and alters our mechanics. Stand tall and ensure your ears, shoulders, hips, and ankles are in alignment.

Second, try to alternate hands where possible. Push with one hand in the center of the stroller handles and use the other arm to swing naturally. This will allow our bodies to go through the natural walking motion, allowing for rotational patterns to occur, and help with force transfer. Place your hands comfortably on the handles without excessive gripping or flexion at the wrist. Push lightly and keep the hands and shoulders fairly relaxed.

Last, adjust handles, positioning, and levers to your body when possible. Many new strollers come with adaptable handles, straps, and levers. Take the time to set up the positioning for your body so that you can keep your shoulders down and relaxed and feel comfortable with the setup and positioning. Think of your ease and comfort when setting things up, because you'll likely be spending years pushing a child or children who will be getting heavier over time. Take the time at the beginning to set things up right and reassess as the children grow. For new parents, taking the new stroller out for a few test drives (perhaps to pick up groceries) may serve as a bridge to help prepare your body for walking while pushing a stroller.

Cross-Training

Walking is without a doubt an excellent physical activity, and we outlined the numerous benefits that walking provides in chapter 1. Adding in variety in walks and training modalities helps to create a more balanced body. Cross-training will ensure we're building capacity, engaging different muscles, loading different areas of the body, preventing overuse injuries, building strength, and ensuring we're able to walk longer, faster, farther, and with more ease.

With over 25 years of experience in sport and fitness, which includes my practice as a Registered Kinesiologist, I have seen overuse injuries from athletes who specialize and specialize young in one sport. Several great athletes grew up playing multiple sports. Sometimes, less is more, and we need to train smarter, not harder. Building tissue tolerance, staying within thresholds, varying activities, and seeking treatment when needed can help athletes remain strong, active, and uninjured.

Find activities you enjoy. As a coach, I would never recommend running if someone didn't enjoy running. Think back to what you enjoyed growing up. When were you the most consistent? What were the parameters where you were the most active and enjoyed it? Sometimes it takes a bit of thinking outside the box, because it doesn't have to be running, biking, swimming, or hiking. Dancing, team sports, skating, tennis or pickleball, group classes, or any activity that elevates your heart rate would be a great cross-training activity, especially if we're adding activities that require different planes of motion. Walking is somewhat linear, and adding a multiplanar activity like pickleball can be a great cross-training option if that's possible to you, understanding that location, equipment, timing, and financial considerations may be limiting factors.

Include some form of strength training in your cross-training programming. Almost all professional coaches would agree on this. Boosting overall strength is important for bone health, muscle health, metabolic health, cognitive health, and more. You'll find specific strength training exercises and recommendations in chapter 9.

Beach

There's nothing like walking on a beach, feeling the warm sand under your feet, the cool breeze on your face, and ocean, lake, or river water splashing at your feet. On your next beach visit, take a stroll along the shore. Walking barefoot, barring any foot discomforts or issues, can be an excellent way to challenge the intrinsic muscles of the feet and train the body in unique ways. You'll experience an earthing or grounding benefit, and adding some movement to a potentially sedentary day adds in some additional physical activity.

These workout suggestions should provide you with options for your future walks. The goal is to include variety and effective, challenging, and fun workouts to target various physiological systems. Progress through the levels as you become more comfortable. The next chapter breaks down specific training plans for 5K, 10K, and half-marathon walking distances.

CHAPTER 12

5K, 10K, and Half-Marathon Training Plans

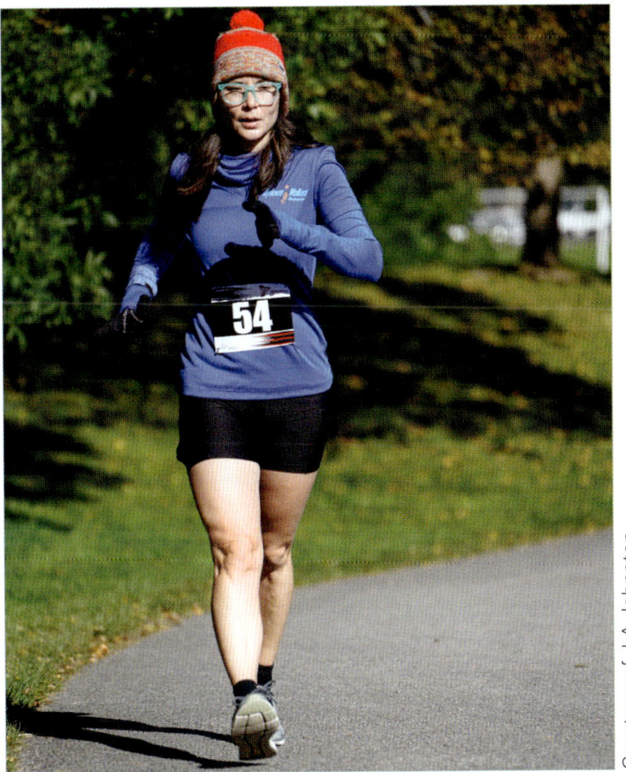

Courtesy of J A Johnston.

This chapter is dedicated to 5K, 10K, and half-marathon training plans. Each plan is broken up into a specific lead-up time, depending on your availability. The longer lead-ups will help you ease and progress to your desired distance with a little more comfort. The more time the body has to adapt, the more adapted and efficient it becomes. The breakdowns will help you to choose what's best for you. If you're fit and active, the shorter lead-ups may work best. If you're someone who does best with slower progressions or are new to a particular distance, the longer lead-ups may be a better starting point for you.

The plans are guidelines, and you're welcome to use them based on your own specific needs. For instance, recommended strength days can fall on other days, depending on your schedule. Separate your two strength days by a walk day, and aim for one longer walk per week, with shorter walks and skill-based walks interspersed. Change the order around if that's best for your training needs. If your weekends are full, your shorter walk can take place on the weekend and your longer walk can occur during the week when you have more time. The distance and time suggestions are just that—suggestions. If you're fatigued and need to adjust, shorten them. If you're energized and strong, ramp them up slightly but aim to stay within the general idea of the progressions. The strength workouts are going to be key to ensure you build capacity for longer distances and time on your feet.

We've outlined one skill-based walk per week (hills or intervals), one longer walk, and two short- to mid-distance walks. The longer- and mid-distance walks are distance-based walks. Shift the distances around slightly but aim to follow the general progression. One walk per week is a time-based walk. This is to shift the focus away from a particular distance and emphasize time on your feet. It can be a slower-paced walk. Get out, enjoy, and don't worry about how far you go. Be consistent with the general plan, and you'll be ready on race day!

5K

The 5K distance is a great starting point for those looking to dip their toes into local races. Or maybe you're just looking to hit that specific distance. The majority of 5K walking races I've participated in have been on a 400-meter track (slightly less than a quarter mile; 12.5 times around); however, I've also walked in 5K races that have meandered through beautiful neighborhoods, historic sights, and waterfront views. Most cities have a plethora of races to choose from with varying causes. Although most races are geared toward runners, most also are walker friendly. Walk your walk and focus on your pace. Give yourself enough time to work up to the full distance. We've outlined 8-week, 10-week, and 12-week training plans, depending on your available lead-up time (tables 12.1-12.3). The final week is a taper week to allow some integration and recovery time in case you're leading up to a race.

TABLE 12.1 8-Week 5K Training Plan

	Monday	Tuesday	Wednesday	Thursday	Friday	Saturday	Sunday
Week 1	Walk 20 min	Strength training	Walk 3 km (1.9 miles)	Hills	Strength training	Walk 3 km (1.9 miles)	Cross-training or day off
Week 2	Walk 22 min	Strength training	Walk 3.5 km (2.2 miles)	Intervals	Strength training	Walk 3.5 km (2.2 miles)	Cross-training or day off
Week 3	Walk 24 min	Strength training	Walk 3.7 km (2.3 miles)	Hills	Strength training	Walk 3.5-4 km (2.2-2.5 miles)	Cross-training or day off
Week 4	Walk 27 min	Strength training	Walk 4 km (2.5 miles)	Intervals	Strength training	Walk 3.5-4 km (2.2-2.5 miles)	Cross-training or day off
Week 5	Walk 30 min	Strength training	Walk 4.2 km (2.6 miles)	Hills	Strength training	Walk 4-4.5 km (2.5-2.8 miles)	Cross-training or day off
Week 6	Walk 30 min	Strength training	Walk 4.5 km (2.8 miles)	Intervals	Strength training	Walk 4.5 km (2.8 miles)	Cross-training or day off
Week 7	Walk 30 min	Strength training	Walk 4 km (2.5 miles)	Hills	Strength training	Walk 5 km (3.1 miles)	Day off
Week 8	Walk 15 min	Strength training	Walk 3 km (1.9 miles)	Intervals	Day off	Walk 3 km (1.9 miles)	Day off

TABLE 12.2 10-Week 5K Training Plan

	Monday	Tuesday	Wednesday	Thursday	Friday	Saturday	Sunday
Week 1	Walk 20 min	Strength training	Walk 3 km (1.9 miles)	Hills	Strength training	Walk 3.5 km (2.2 miles)	Cross-training or day off
Week 2	Walk 22 min	Strength training	Walk 3 km (1.9 miles)	Intervals	Strength training	Walk 3.5 km (2.2 miles)	Cross-training or day off
Week 3	Walk 24 min	Strength training	Walk 3.5 km (2.2 miles)	Hills	Strength training	Walk 3.5-4 km (2.2-2.5 miles)	Cross-training or day off
Week 4	Walk 26 min	Strength training	Walk 3.7 km (2.3 miles)	Intervals	Strength training	Walk 3.5-4 km (2.2-2.5 miles)	Cross-training or day off
Week 5	Walk 28 min	Strength training	Walk 4 km (2.5 miles)	Hills	Strength training	Walk 4 km (2.5 miles)	Cross-training or day off
Week 6	Walk 30 min	Strength training	Walk 4.2 km (2.6 miles)	Intervals	Strength training	Walk 4 km (2.5 miles)	Cross-training or day off
Week 7	Walk 30 min	Strength training	Walk 4.5 km (2.8 miles)	Hills	Strength training	Walk 4-4.5 km (2.5-2.8 miles)	Cross-training or day off
Week 8	Walk 25 min	Strength training	Walk 4 km (2.5 miles)	Intervals	Strength training	Walk 4.5 km (2.8 miles)	Cross-training or day off
Week 9	Walk 20 min	Strength training	Walk 3 km (1.9 miles)	Hills	Strength training	Walk 5 km (3.1 miles)	Day off
Week 10	Walk 15 min	Strength training	Walk 2 km (1.2 miles)	Intervals	Day off	Walk 3.5 km (2.2 miles)	Day off

TABLE 12.3 12-Week 5K Training Plan

	Monday	Tuesday	Wednesday	Thursday	Friday	Saturday	Sunday
Week 1	Walk 20 min	Strength training	Walk 2.5 km (1.5 miles)	Hills	Strength training	Walk 3 km (1.9 miles)	Cross-training or day off
Week 2	Walk 20 min	Strength training	Walk 2.5 km (1.5 miles)	Intervals	Strength training	Walk 3-3.5 km (1.9-2.2 miles)	Cross-training or day off
Week 3	Walk 22 min	Strength training	Walk 3 km (1.9 miles)	Hills	Strength training	Walk 3.5 km (2.2 miles)	Cross-training or day off
Week 4	Walk 22 min	Strength training	Walk 3 km (1.9 miles)	Intervals	Strength training	Walk 3.5-4 km (2.2-2.5 miles)	Cross-training or day off
Week 5	Walk 24 min	Strength training	Walk 3.5 km (2.2 miles)	Hills	Strength training	Walk 4 km (2.5 miles)	Cross-training or day off
Week 6	Walk 25 min	Strength training	Walk 3.5 km (2.2 miles)	Intervals	Strength training	Walk 4-4.5 km (2.5-2.8 miles)	Cross-training or day off
Week 7	Walk 25 min	Strength training	Walk 4 km (2.5 miles)	Hills	Strength training	Walk 4.5 km (2.8 miles)	Cross-training or day off
Week 8	Walk 28 min	Strength training	Walk 4 km (2.5 miles)	Intervals	Strength training	Walk 4.5 km (2.8 miles)	Cross-training or day off
Week 9	Walk 30 min	Strength training	Walk 4.5 km (2.8 miles)	Hills	Strength training	Walk 4.5-4.8 km (2.8-3 miles)	Cross-training or day off
Week 10	Walk 30 min	Strength training	Walk 4 km (2.5 miles)	Intervals	Strength training	Walk 4.8 km (3 miles)	Cross-training or day off
Week 11	Walk 25 min	Strength training	Walk 3 km (1.9 miles)	Hills	Strength training	Walk 5 km (3.1 miles)	Day off
Week 12	Walk 15 min	Strength training	Walk 2 km (1.2 miles)	Intervals	Day off	Walk 3.5 km (2.2 miles)	Day off

10K

The 10K walk is certainly a more challenging walk. It's a great option for those who find the 5K distance easy, or for anyone wanting to build up to a half-marathon distance. It's not an easy one to work up to, and you'll want a good base with lots of longer walks and skill-based walks under your belt. We've included 10-, 12-, and 16-week buildup plans (tables 12.4-12.6), but feel free to repeat weeks and take longer to work your way up if that's best for you.

TABLE 12.4 10-Week 10K Training Plan

	Monday	Tuesday	Wednesday	Thursday	Friday	Saturday	Sunday
Week 1	Walk 30 min	Strength training	Walk 4 km (2.5 miles)	Hills	Strength training	Walk 6 km (3.7 miles)	Cross-training or day off
Week 2	Walk 35 min	Strength training	Walk 4.5 km (2.8 miles)	Intervals	Strength training	Walk 6.5 km (4 miles)	Cross-training or day off
Week 3	Walk 35 min	Strength training	Walk 4.5 km (2.8 miles)	Hills	Strength training	Walk 7 km (4.3 miles)	Cross-training or day off
Week 4	Walk 40 min	Strength training	Walk 5 km (3.1 miles)	Intervals	Strength training	Walk 7.5 km (4.7 miles)	Cross-training or day off
Week 5	Walk 40 min	Strength training	Walk 5 km (3.1 miles)	Hills	Strength training	Walk 8 km (5 miles)	Cross-training or day off
Week 6	Walk 45 min	Strength training	Walk 5.5 km (3.4 miles)	Intervals	Strength training	Walk 8.5 km (5.3 miles)	Cross-training or day off
Week 7	Walk 45 min	Strength training	Walk 5.5 km (3.4 miles)	Hills	Strength training	Walk 9 km (5.6 miles)	Cross-training or day off
Week 8	Walk 50 min	Strength training	Walk 6 km (3.7 miles)	Intervals	Strength training	Walk 9.5 km (5.9 miles)	Cross-training or day off
Week 9	Walk 50 min	Strength training	Walk 6.5 km (4 miles)	Hills	Strength training	Walk 10 km (6.2 miles)	Day off
Week 10	Walk 30 min	Strength training	Walk 2 km (1.2 miles)	Intervals	Day off	Walk 5 km (3.1 miles)	Day off

TABLE 12.5 12-Week 10K Training Plan

	Monday	Tuesday	Wednesday	Thursday	Friday	Saturday	Sunday
Week 1	Walk 30 min	Strength training	Walk 4 km (2.5 miles)	Hills	Strength training	Walk 6 km (3.7 miles)	Cross-training or day off
Week 2	Walk 35 min	Strength training	Walk 4 km (2.5 miles)	Intervals	Strength training	Walk 6.5 km (4 miles)	Cross-training or day off
Week 3	Walk 35 min	Strength training	Walk 4.5 km (2.8 miles)	Hills	Strength training	Walk 7 km (4.3 miles)	Cross-training or day off
Week 4	Walk 40 min	Strength training	Walk 4.5 km (2.8 miles)	Intervals	Strength training	Walk 7.5 km (4.7 miles)	Cross-training or day off
Week 5	Walk 40 min	Strength training	Walk 5 km (3.1 miles)	Hills	Strength training	Walk 8 km (5 miles)	Cross-training or day off
Week 6	Walk 45 min	Strength training	Walk 5 km (3.1 miles)	Intervals	Strength training	Walk 8.5 km (5.2 miles)	Cross-training or day off
Week 7	Walk 45 min	Strength training	Walk 5.5 km (3.4 miles)	Hills	Strength training	Walk 8.5 km (5.2 miles)	Cross-training or day off
Week 8	Walk 50 min	Strength training	Walk 5.5 km (3.4 miles)	Intervals	Strength training	Walk 9 km (5.6 miles)	Cross-training or day off
Week 9	Walk 50 min	Strength training	Walk 6 km (3.7 miles)	Hills	Strength training	Walk 9 km (5.6 miles)	Cross-training or day off
Week 10	Walk 55 min	Strength training	Walk 6 km (3.7 miles)	Intervals	Strength training	Walk 9.5 km (5.9 miles)	Cross-training or day off
Week 11	Walk 55 min	Strength training	Walk 6.5 km (4 miles)	Hills	Strength training	Walk 10 km (6.2 miles)	Day off
Week 12	Walk 30 min	Strength training	Walk 7 km (4.3 miles)	Intervals	Day off	Walk 5 km (3.1 miles)	Day off

TABLE 12.6 16-Week 10K Training Plan

	Monday	Tuesday	Wednesday	Thursday	Friday	Saturday	Sunday
Week 1	Walk 30 min	Strength training	Walk 4 km (2.5 miles)	Hills	Strength training	Walk 6 km (3.7 miles)	Cross-training or day off
Week 2	Walk 30 min	Strength training	Walk 4 km (2.5 miles)	Intervals	Strength training	Walk 6 km (3.7 miles)	Cross-training or day off
Week 3	Walk 35 min	Strength training	Walk 4.5 km (2.8 miles)	Hills	Strength training	Walk 6.5 km (4 miles)	Cross-training or day off
Week 4	Walk 35 min	Strength training	Walk 4.5 km (2.8 miles)	Intervals	Strength training	Walk 6.5 km (4 miles)	Cross-training or day off
Week 5	Walk 40 min	Strength training	Walk 5 km (3.1 miles)	Hills	Strength training	Walk 7 km (4.3 miles)	Cross-training or day off
Week 6	Walk 40 min	Strength training	Walk 5 km (3.1 miles)	Intervals	Strength training	Walk 7 km (4.3 miles)	Cross-training or day off
Week 7	Walk 45 min	Strength training	Walk 5.5 km (3.4 miles)	Hills	Strength training	Walk 7.5 km (4.7 miles)	Cross-training or day off
Week 8	Walk 45 min	Strength training	Walk 5.5 km (3.4 miles)	Intervals	Strength training	Walk 7.5 km (4.7 miles)	Cross-training or day off
Week 9	Walk 50 min	Strength training	Walk 6 km (3.7 miles)	Hills	Strength training	Walk 8 km (5 miles)	Cross-training or day off
Week 10	Walk 50 min	Strength training	Walk 6 km (3.7 miles)	Intervals	Strength training	Walk 8 km (5 miles)	Cross-training or day off
Week 11	Walk 55 min	Strength training	Walk 6.5 km (4 miles)	Hills	Strength training	Walk 8.5 km (5.2 miles)	Cross-training or day off
Week 12	Walk 55 min	Strength training	Walk 6.5 km (4 miles)	Intervals	Strength training	Walk 9 km (5.6 miles)	Cross-training or day off
Week 13	Walk 60 min	Strength training	Walk 7 km (4.3 miles)	Hills	Strength training	Walk 9 km (5.6 miles)	Cross-training or day off
Week 14	Walk 60 min	Strength training	Walk 7 km (4.3 miles)	Intervals	Strength training	Walk 9.5 km (5.9 miles)	Cross-training or day off
Week 15	Walk 60 min	Strength training	Walk 7 km (4.3 miles)	Hills	Strength training	Walk 10 km (6.2 miles)	Day off
Week 16	Walk 30 min	Strength training	Walk 4 km (2.5 miles)	Intervals	Day off	Walk 5 km (3.1 miles)	Day off

Half-Marathon

The half-marathon distance is no easy feat. However, for avid walkers, it's a manageable distance for anyone who is well conditioned and experienced. The distance is challenging without rendering most participants overly depleted. We have provided 12- and 16-week lead-up plans (tables 12.7-12.8), but if you're newer or need more time, repeat weeks

TABLE 12.7 12-Week Half-Marathon Training Plan

	Monday	Tuesday	Wednesday	Thursday	Friday	Saturday	Sunday
Week 1	Walk 30 min	Strength training	Walk 5 km (3.1 miles)	Hills	Strength training	Walk 10 km (6.2 miles)	Cross-training or day off
Week 2	Walk 30 min	Strength training	Walk 6 km (3.7 miles)	Intervals	Strength training	Walk 11 km (6.8 miles)	Cross-training or day off
Week 3	Walk 35 min	Strength training	Walk 7 km (4.3 miles)	Hills	Strength training	Walk 12 km (7.5 miles)	Cross-training or day off
Week 4	Walk 40 min	Strength training	Walk 7 km (4.3 miles)	Intervals	Strength training	Walk 13 km (8.1 miles)	Cross-training or day off
Week 5	Walk 40 min	Strength training	Walk 8 km (5 miles)	Hills	Strength training	Walk 14 km (8.7 miles)	Cross-training or day off
Week 6	Walk 45 min	Strength training	Walk 8 km (5 miles)	Intervals	Strength training	Walk 15 km (9.3 miles)	Cross-training or day off
Week 7	Walk 45 min	Strength training	Walk 9 km (5.6 miles)	Hills	Strength training	Walk 16 km (9.9 miles)	Cross-training or day off
Week 8	Walk 50 min	Strength training	Walk 9 km (5.6 miles)	Intervals	Strength training	Walk 17 km (10.6 miles)	Cross-training or day off
Week 9	Walk 50 min	Strength training	Walk 10 km (6.2 miles)	Hills	Strength training	Walk 18 km (11.2 miles)	Cross-training or day off
Week 10	Walk 55 min	Strength training	Walk 10 km (6.2 miles)	Intervals	Strength training	Walk 20 km (12.4 miles)	Cross-training or day off
Week 11	Walk 60 min	Strength training	Walk 10 km (6.2 miles)	Hills	Strength training	Walk 21 km (13 miles)	Day off
Week 12	Walk 60 min	Strength training	Walk 5 km (3.1 miles)	Intervals	Day off	Walk 8 km (5 miles)	Day off

TABLE 12.8 16-Week Half-Marathon Training Plan

	Monday	Tuesday	Wednesday	Thursday	Friday	Saturday	Sunday
Week 1	Walk 30 min	Strength training	Walk 5 km (3.1 miles)	Hills	Strength training	Walk 10 km (6.2 miles)	Cross-training or day off
Week 2	Walk 30 min	Strength training	Walk 5 km (3.1 miles)	Intervals	Strength training	Walk 11 km (6.8 miles)	Cross-training or day off
Week 3	Walk 35 min	Strength training	Walk 6 km 3.7 miles)	Hills	Strength training	Walk 12 km (7.5 miles)	Cross-training or day off
Week 4	Walk 35 min	Strength training	Walk 6 km (3.7 miles)	Intervals	Strength training	Walk 13 km (8.1 miles)	Cross-training or day off
Week 5	Walk 40 min	Strength training	Walk 7 km (4.3 miles)	Hills	Strength training	Walk 14 km (8.7 miles)	Cross-training or day off
Week 6	Walk 40 min	Strength training	Walk 7 km (4.3 miles)	Intervals	Strength training	Walk 15 km (9.3 miles)	Cross-training or day off
Week 7	Walk 45 min	Strength training	Walk 8 km (5 miles)	Hills	Strength training	Walk 15 km (9.3 miles)	Cross-training or day off
Week 8	Walk 45 min	Strength training	Walk 8 km (5 miles)	Intervals	Strength training	Walk 16 km (9.9 miles)	Cross-training or day off
Week 9	Walk 45 min	Strength training	Walk 9 km (5.6 miles)	Hills	Strength training	Walk 16 km (10 miles)	Cross-training or day off
Week 10	Walk 45 min	Strength training	Walk 9 km (5.6 miles)	Intervals	Strength training	Walk 17 km (10.6 miles)	Cross-training or day off
Week 11	Walk 50 min	Strength training	Walk 10 km (6.2 miles)	Hills	Strength training	Walk 17 km (10.6 miles)	Cross-training or day off
Week 12	Walk 50 min	Strength training	Walk 10 km (6.2 miles)	Intervals	Strength training	Walk 19 km (11.8 miles)	Cross-training or day off
Week 13	Walk 55 min	Strength training	Walk 9 km (5.6 miles)	Hills	Strength training	Walk 19 km (11.8 miles)	Cross-training or day off
Week 14	Walk 55 min	Strength training	Walk 8 km (5 miles)	Intervals	Strength training	Walk 20 km (12.4 miles)	Cross-training or day off
Week 15	Walk 60 min	Strength training	Walk 7 km (4.3 miles)	Hills	Strength training	Walk 21 km (13 miles)	Day off
Week 16	Walk 30 min	Strength training	Walk 6 km (3.7 miles)	Intervals	Day off	Walk 10 km (6.2 miles)	Day off

to build up progressively and comfortably. Your strength days will be important to build tissue tolerance and capacity for your longer walks and for life. Most walkers prefer the shorter distance, and for those attempting the half-marathon, I commend you and encourage you to stay consistent and take breaks when needed.

We hope these training plans provide some guidance, structure, and assistance to help you build your best walking routine and get the most out of each and every one of your walks. We hope you continue to walk for your body, brain, heart, and bones, and for your overall fitness, health, and wellness. Health is wealth, and walking invests in your body as surely as putting money in a mutual fund invests in your future. Stay consistent, add variety, warm up, cool down, strengthen, and keep walking!

REFERENCES

CHAPTER 1

Bell SL, Audrey S, Gunnell D, Cooper A, and Campbell R. 2019. "The Relationship Between Physical Activity, Mental Wellbeing and Symptoms of Mental Health Disorder in Adolescents: A Cohort Study." *International Journal of Behavioural Nutrition and Physical Activity* 16: 138. https://doi.org/10.1186/s12966-019-0901-7.

Chastin SFM, Abaraogu U, Bourgois JG, Dall PM, Darnborough J, Duncan E, Dumortier J, Jimenez-Pavon D, McParland J, Roberts NJ, and Hamer M. 2021. "Effects of Regular Physical Activity on the Immune System, Vaccination and Risk of Community-Acquired Infectious Disease in the General Population: Systematic Review and Meta-Analysis." *Sports Medicine* 51, no. 8: 1673-1686.

Chekroud SR, Gueorguieva R, Zheutlin AB, Paulus M, Krumholz HM, Krystal JH, and Chekroud AM. 2018. "Association Between Physical Exercise and Mental Health in 1.2 Million Individuals in the USA Between 2011 and 2015: A Cross-Sectional Study." *Lancet Psychiatry*. Sep;5(9):739-746. https://doi.org/10.1016/S2215-0366(18)30227-X. Epub 2018 Aug 8. PMID: 30099000.

Chevalier G, Sinatra ST, Oschman JL, Sokal K, and Sokal P. 2012. "Earthing: Health Implications of Reconnecting the Human Body to the Earth's Surface Electrons." *Journal of Environmental and Public Health*. Jan 12;2012:291541. https://doi.org/10.1155/2012/291541.

Coulson JC, McKenna J, and Field M. 2008. "Exercising at Work and Self-Reported Work Performance." *International Journal of Workplace Health Management* 1, no. 3: 176-197. https://doi.org/10.1108/17538350810926534.

Dumurgier J, Elbaz A, Ducimetière P, Tavernier B, Alpérovitch A, and Tzourio C. 2009. "Slow Walking Speed and Cardiovascular Death in Well Functioning Older Adults: Prospective Cohort Study." *BMJ* 2009;339:b4460.

Fujita K, Takahashi H, Miura C, Ohkubo T, Sato Y, Ugajin T, Kurashima K, Tsubono Y, Tsuji I, Fukao A, and Hisamichi S. 2004. "Walking and Mortality in Japan: The Miyagi Cohort Study." *Journal of Epidemiology*. Feb;14 Suppl 1(Suppl I):S26-32. https://doi.org/10.2188/jea.14.s26.

Garcia L, Pearce M, Abbas A, Mok A, Strain T, Ali S, Crippa A, Dempsey PC, Golubic R, Kelly P, Laird Y, McNamara E, Moore S, de Sa TH, Smith AD, Wijndaele K, and Woodcock J, Brage S. 2023. "Non-Occupational Physical Activity and Risk of Cardiovascular Disease, Cancer and Mortality Outcomes: A Dose-Response Meta-Analysis of Large Prospective Studies." *British Journal of Sports Medicine*. Aug;57(15):979-989. https://doi.org/10.1136/bjsports-2022-105669.

Hamer M, Stamatakis E, and Steptoe A. 2008. "Dose-Response Relationship Between Physical Activity and Mental Health: The Scottish Health Survey." *British Journal of Sports Medicine*. 43(14):1111-4. https://doi.org/10.1136/bjsm.2008.046243.

Hanson S, and Jones A. 2015. "Is There Evidence That Walking Groups Have Health Benefits? A Systematic Review and Meta-Analysis." *British Journal of Sports Medicine*. Jun;49(11):710-715. https://doi.org/10.1136/bjsports-2014-094157. Epub 2015 Jan 19. PMID: 25601182; PMCID: PMC4453623.

Hardman AE, Jones PR, Norgan NG, and Hudson A. 1992. "Brisk Walking Improves Endurance Fitness Without Changing Body Fatness in Previously Sedentary Women."

European Journal of Applied Physiology and Occupational Physiology. 65(4):354-359. https://doi.org/10.1007/BF00868140. PMID: 1425636.

Hosseini-Asl MK, Taherifard E, and Mousavi MR. 2021. "The Effect of a Short-Term Physical Activity After Meals on Gastrointestinal Symptoms in Individuals With Functional Abdominal Bloating: A Randomized Clinical Trial." *Gastroenterology and Hepatology: From Bed to Bench*. Winter;14(1):59-66.

Inoue K, Tsugawa Y, Mayeda ER, and Ritz B. 2023. "Association of Daily Step Patterns with Mortality in US Adults." *JAMA Network Open*. Mar 1;6(3):e235174. https://doi.org/10.1001/jamanetworkopen.2023.5174.

Jayedi A, Gohari A, and Shab-Bidar S. 2022. "Daily Step Count and All-Cause Mortality: A Dose–Response Meta-Analysis of Prospective Cohort Studies." *Journal of Sports Medicine* 52, no. 1: 89-99.

Jayedi A, Zargar M, Emadi A, and Aune, D. 2024. "Walking Speed and the Risk of Type 2 Diabetes: A Systematic Review and Meta-Analysis." *British Journal of Sports Medicine*. Mar 13;58(6):334-342. https://doi.org/10.1136/bjsports-2023-107336.

Jones ML, Evans N, Tefertiller C, Backus D, Sweatman M, Tansey K, and Morrison S. 2014. "Activity-Based Therapy for Recovery of Walking in Individuals With Chronic Spinal Cord Injury: Results From a Randomized Clinical Trial." *Archives of Physical Medicine and Rehabilitation* 95, no. 12, 2239-2246.e2.

Krall EA, and Dawson-Hughes B. 1994. "Walking Is Related to Bone Density and Rates of Bone Loss." *American Journal of Medicine*. Jan;96(1):20-26. https://doi.org/10.1016/0002-9343(94)90111-2. PMID: 8304358.

Lan YS, and Feng YJ. 2022. "The Volume of Brisk Walking Is the Key Determinant of BMD Improvement in Premenopausal Women." *PLOS ONE*. Mar 16;17(3):e0265250. https://doi.org/10.1371/journal.pone.0265250.

Mahindru A, Patil P, and Agrawal V. 2023. "Role of Physical Activity on Mental Health and Well-Being: A Review." *Cureus*. Jan 7;15(1):e33475. https://doi.org/10.7759/cureus.33475.

Manson JE, Hu FB, Rich-Edwards JW, Colditz GA, Stampfer MJ, Willet WC, Speizer FE, and Hennekens CH. 1999. "A Prospective Study of Walking as Compared With Vigorous Exercise in the Prevention of Coronary Heart Disease in Women." New England Journal of Medicine. 341:650-658. https://doi.org/10.1056/NEJM199908263410904.

Mau M, Aaby A, Klausen SH, and Roessler KK. 2021. "Are Long-Distance Walks Therapeutic? A Systematic Scoping Review of the Conceptualization of Long-Distance Walking and Its Relation to Mental Health." *International Journal of Environmental Research and Public Health*. Jul 21;18(15):7741. https://doi.org/10.3390/ijerph18157741.

The Mayo Clinic. 2023. "Depression and Anxiety: Exercise Eases Symptoms." https://www.mayoclinic.org/diseases-conditions/depression/in-depth/depression-and-exercise/art-20046495.

Moore SC, Lee IM, Weiderpass E, Campbell PT, Sampson JN, Kitahara CM, Keadle SK, Arem H, Berrington de Gonzalez A, Hartge P, Adami HO, Blair CK, Borch KB, Boyd E, Check DP, Fournier A, Freedman ND, Gunter M, Johannson M, Khaw KT, Linet MS, Orsini N, Park Y, Riboli E, Robien K, Schairer C, Sesso H, Spriggs M, Van Dusen R, Wolk A, Matthews CE, and Patel AV. Association of Leisure-Time Physical Activity With Risk of 26 Types of Cancer in 1.44 Million Adults. *JAMA Intern Med*. 2016 Jun 1;176(6):816-25. https://doi.org/10.1001/jamainternmed.2016.1548. PMID: 27183032; PMCID: PMC5812009.

National Geographic. 2019. "The Secret to Mindful Travel? A Walk in the Woods." https://www.nationalgeographic.com/travel/article/forest-bathing-nature-walk-health.

Nieman DC, Henson DA, Austin MD, and Sha W. 2011. "Upper Respiratory Tract Infection Is Reduced in Physically Fit and Active Adults." *British Journal of Sports Medicine* 45:987-992.

Oppezzo M, and Schwartz DL. 2014. "Give Your Ideas Some Legs: The Positive Effect of Walking on Creative Thinking." *Journal of Experimental Psychology: Learning, Memory and Cognition*. Jul;40(4):1142-52. https://doi.org/10.1037/a0036577. Epub 2014 Apr 21. PMID: 24749966.

Paluch AE, Bajpai S, Ballin M, Bassett DR, Buford TW, Carnethon MR, Chernofsky A, Dooley EE, Ekelund U, Evenson KR, Galuska DA, Jefferis BJ, Kong L, Kraus WE, Larson MG, Lee IM, Matthews CE, Newton RL Jr, Nordström A, Nordström P, Palta P, Patel AV, Pettee Gabriel K, Pieper CF, Pompeii L, Rees-Punia E, Spartano NL, Vasan RS, Whincup PH, Yang S, and Fulton JE; Steps for Health Collaborative. 2023. "Prospective Association of Daily Steps With Cardiovascular Disease: A Harmonized Meta-Analysis." *Circulation*. 147(2):122-131. https://doi.org/10.1161/CIRCULATIONAHA.122.061288.

Peachman RR. 2022. "Will Exercising With a Cold Make You Sicker?" *New York Times*, December 6, 2022, https://www.nytimes.com/2022/11/29/well/move/exercise-sick-cold.html.

Reynolds AN, and Venn BJ. 2018. "The Timing of Activity After Eating Affects the Glycaemic Response of Healthy Adults: A Randomised Controlled Trial." *Nutrients*. Nov 13;10(11):1743. https://doi.org/10.3390/nu10111743.

Rodríguez-Romo G, Acebes-Sánchez J, García-Merino S, Garrido-Muñoz M, Blanco-García C, and Diez-Vega I. 2022. "Physical Activity and Mental Health in Undergraduate Students." *International Journal of Environmental Research and Public Health*. Dec 23;20(1):195. https://doi.org/10.3390/ijerph20010195.

Sabiston CM, Jewett R, Ashdown-Franks G, Belanger M, Brunet J, O'Loughlin E, and O'Loughlin J. 2016. Number of Years of Team and Individual Sport Participation During Adolescence and Depressive Symptoms in Early Adulthood. *J Sport Exerc Psychol*. 2016 Feb;38(1):105-10. https://doi.org/10.1123/jsep.2015-0175. PMID: 27018562.

Sakuragi S, and Sugiyama Y. 2006. "Effects of Daily Walking on Subjective Symptoms, Mood and Autonomic Nervous Function." *Journal of Physiological Anthropology*. Jul;25(4):281-9. https://doi.org/10.2114/jpa2.25.281.

Sheng M, Yang J, Bao M, Chen T, Cai R, Zhang N, Chen H, Liu M, Wu X, Zhang B, Liu Y, and Chao J. 2021. "The Relationships Between Step Count and All-Cause Mortality and Cardiovascular Events: A Dose-Response Meta-Analysis." *Journal of Sport and Health Science*. Dec;10(6):620-628. https://doi.org/10.1016/j.jshs.2021.09.004.

Siddarth P, Rahi B, Emerson ND, Burggren AC, Miller KJ, Bookheimer S, Lavretsky H, Dobkin B, Small G, and Merrill DA. 2018. "Physical Activity and Hippocampal Sub-Region Structure in Older Adults With Memory Complaints." *Journal of Alzheimer's Disease*. 61(3):1089-1096. https://doi.org/10.3233/JAD-170586.

Singh B, Olds T, Curtis R, Dumuid D, Virgara R, Watson A, Szeto K, O'Connor E, Ferguson T, Eglitis E, Miatke A, Simpson CEM, and Maher C. 2023. "Effectiveness of Physical Activity Interventions for Improving Depression, Anxiety and Distress: An Overview of Systematic Reviews." *British Journal of Sports Medicine*. 57:1203-1209.

Steinhilber B. "Why Walking Is the Most Underrated Form of Exercise." NBC, September 2, 2017. https://www.nbcnews.com/better/health/why-walking-most-underrated-form-exercise-ncna797271.

Stubbs B, Vancampfort D, Smith L, Rosenbaum S, Schuch F, and Firth J. 2018. "Physical Activity and Mental Health." *The Lancet Psychiatry* 5, no. 11 (Sept.): P873. https://doi.org/https://doi.org/10.1016/S2215-0366(18)30343-2.

University of South Australia. 2023. "Exercise More Effective Than Medicines to Manage Mental Health, Study Shows." ScienceDaily. www.sciencedaily.com/releases/2023/02/230223193417.htm (accessed December 26, 2023).

White MP, Alcock I, Grellier J, Wheeler BW, Hartig T, Warber SL, Bone A, Depledge MH, and Fleming LE, 2019. "Spending at Least 120 Minutes a Week in Nature Is Associated With Good Health and Wellbeing." *Scientific Reports* 9 (June): 7730.

Yamada M, Nishiguchi S, Fukutani N, Aoyama T, and Arai H. 2015. "Mail-Based Intervention for Sarcopenia Prevention Increased Anabolic Hormone and Skeletal Muscle Mass in Community-Dwelling Japanese Older Adults: The INE (Intervention by Nutrition and Exercise) Study." *Journal of the American Medical Directors Association*. Aug 1;16(8):654-60. https://doi.org/10.1016/j.jamda.2015.02.017.

Zaccardi F, Franks PW, Dudbridge F, Davies MJ, Khunti K, and Yates T. 2021. "Mortality Risk Comparing Walking Pace to Handgrip Strength and a Healthy Lifestyle: A UK Biobank Study." *European Journal of Preventive Cardiology*. Jul 10;28(7):704-712. https://doi.org/10.1177/2047487319885041.

CHAPTER 2

Chen YC, Walhin JP, Hengist A, Gonzalez JT, Betts JA, and Thompson D. Interrupting Prolonged Sitting With Intermittent Walking Increases Postprandial Gut Hormone Responses. *Med Sci Sports Exerc*. 2022 Jul 1;54(7):1183-1189. https://doi.org/10.1249/MSS.0000000000002903.

Kamiya K, Masuda T, Tanaka S, Hamazaki N, Matsue Y, Mezzani A, Matsuzawa R, Nozaki K, Maekawa E, Noda C, Yamaoka-Tojo M, Arai Y, Matsunaga A, Izumi T, and Ako J. Quadriceps Strength as a Predictor of Mortality in Coronary Artery Disease. *Am J Med*. 2015 Nov;128(11):1212-9. https://doi.org/10.1016/j.amjmed.2015.06.035.

Prasetyo M, Nindita N, Nyoman Murdana I, Prihartono J, and Setiawan SI. 2020. Computed Tomography Evaluation of Fat Infiltration Ratio of the Multifidus Muscle in Chronic Low Back Pain Patients. *European J Radiology Open* 7 (2020): 100293. https://doi.org/10.1016/j.ejro.2020.100293.

Yamada M, Nishiguchi S, Fukutani N, Aoyama T, and Arai H. Mail-Based Intervention for Sarcopenia Prevention Increased Anabolic Hormone and Skeletal Muscle Mass in Community-Dwelling Japanese Older Adults: The INE (Intervention by Nutrition and Exercise) Study. *J Am Med Dir Assoc*. 2015 Aug 1;16(8):654-60. https://doi.org/10.1016/j.jamda.2015.02.017.

CHAPTER 3

Bento G, and Dias G. The Importance of Outdoor Play for Young Children's Healthy Development. *Porto Biomed J*. 2017 Sep-Oct;2(5):157-160. https://doi.org/10.1016/j.pbj.2017.03.003. Epub 2017 Apr 6. PMID: 32258612; PMCID: PMC6806863.

Curtis R, Willems C, Paoletti P, and D'Août K. Daily Activity in Minimal Footwear Increases Foot Strength. *Sci Rep*. 2021 Sep 20;11(1):18648. https://doi.org/10.1038/s41598-021-98070-0. PMID: 34545114; PMCID: PMC8452613.

DeVille NV, Tomasso LP, Stoddard OP, Wilt GE, Horton TH, Wolf KL, Brymer E, Kahn PH Jr, and James P. Time Spent in Nature Is Associated With Increased Pro-Environmental Attitudes and Behaviors. *Int J Environ Res Public Health*. 2021 Jul 14;18(14):7498. https://doi.org/10.3390/ijerph18147498. PMID: 34299948; PMCID: PMC8305895.

Ferguson T, Olds T, Curtis R, Blake H, Crozier AJ, Dankiw K, Dumuid D, Kasai D, O'Connor E, Virgara R, and Maher C. Effectiveness of Wearable Activity Trackers to Increase Physical Activity and Improve Health: A Systematic Review of Systematic Reviews and Meta-Analyses. *Lancet Digit Health*. 2022 Aug;4(8):e615-e626. https://doi.org/10.1016/S2589-7500(22)00111-X. PMID: 35868813.

Franklin S, Grey MJ, Heneghan N, Bowen L, and Li FX. Barefoot vs Common Footwear: A Systematic Review of the Kinematic, Kinetic and Muscle Activity Differences During Walking. *Gait Posture*. 2015 Sep;42(3):230-9. https://doi.org/10.1016/j.gaitpost.2015.05.019. Epub 2015 Jun 3. PMID: 26220400.

Gottschall JS, and Nichols TR. Neuromuscular Strategies for the Transitions Between Level and Hill Surfaces During Walking. *Philos Trans R Soc Lond B Biol Sci*. 2011 May 27;366(1570):1565-79. https://doi.org/10.1098/rstb.2010.0355. PMID: 21502127; PMCID: PMC3130452.

Leicht AS, and Crowther RG. Pedometer Accuracy During Walking Over Different Surfaces. *Med Sci Sports Exerc*. 2007 Oct;39(10):1847-50. https://doi.org/10.1249/mss.0b013e3181405b9f. Erratum in: Med Sci Sports Exerc. 2008 Feb;40(2):400. PMID: 17909414.

Lejeune TM, Willems PA, and Heglund NC. Mechanics and Energetics of Human Locomotion on Sand. *J Exp Biol*. 1998 Jul;201(Pt 13):2071-80. https://doi.org/10.1242/jeb.201.13.2071. PMID: 9622579.

Oppezzo M, and Schwartz DL. Give Your Ideas Some Legs: The Positive Effect of Walking on Creative Thinking. *J Exp Psychol Learn Mem Cogn*. 2014 Jul;40(4):1142-52. https://doi.org/10.1037/a0036577. Epub 2014 Apr 21. PMID: 24749966.

Thomas NDA, Gardiner JD, Crompton RH, and Lawson R. Physical and Perceptual Measures of Walking Surface Complexity Strongly Predict Gait and Gaze Behaviour. *Hum Mov Sci*. 2020 Jun;71:102615. https://doi.org/10.1016/j.humov.2020.102615. Epub 2020 Mar 28. PMID: 32452433.

CHAPTER 4

Fincham GW, Strauss C, Montero-Marin J, and Cavanagh K. Effect of Breathwork on Stress and Mental Health: A Meta-Analysis of Randomised-Controlled Trials. *Sci Rep* 13 (2023): 432. https://doi.org/10.1038/s41598-022-27247-y.

Kim D, Cho M, Park Y, and Yang Y. Effect of an Exercise Program for Posture Correction on Musculoskeletal Pain. *J Phys Ther Sci*. 2015 Jun;27(6):1791-4. https://doi.org/10.1589/jpts.27.1791. Epub 2015 Jun 30. PMID: 26180322; PMCID: PMC4499985.

Zaccaro A, Piarulli A, Laurino M, Garbella E, Menicucci D, Neri B, and Gemignani A. How Breath-Control Can Change Your Life: A Systematic Review on Psycho-Physiological Correlates of Slow Breathing. *Front Hum Neurosci*. 2018 Sep 7;12:353. https://doi.org/10.3389/fnhum.2018.00353. PMID: 30245619; PMCID: PMC6137615.

CHAPTER 5

Alexander RM. Tendon Elasticity and Muscle Function. *Comp Biochem Physiol A Mol Integr Physiol*. 2002 Dec;133(4):1001-11. https://doi.org/10.1016/s1095-6433(02)00143-5. PMID: 12485689.

Ardestani MM, Ferrigno C, Maazen M, and Wimmer MA. From Normal to Fast Walking: Impact of Cadence and Stride Length on Lower Extremity Joint Moments. *Journal of Gait and Posture* 46 (May 2016): 118-125. https://doi.org/10.1016/j.gaitpost.2016.02.005.

Del Pozo Cruz B, Ahmadi MN, Lee IM, and Stamatakis E. Prospective Associations of Daily Step Counts and Intensity With Cancer and Cardiovascular Disease Incidence and Mortality and All-Cause Mortality. *JAMA Intern Med*. 2022 Nov 1;182(11):1139-1148. https://doi.org/10.1001/jamainternmed.2022.4000. PMID: 36094529; PMCID: PMC9468953.

Gill N, O'Leary T, Roberts A, Liu A, Roerdink M, Greeves J, and Jones R. Enforcing Walking Speed and Step-Length Affects Joint Kinematics and Kinetics in Male and Female Healthy Adults. *Gait Posture*. 2023 Jun;103:223-228. https://doi.org/10.1016/j.gaitpost.2023.05.025. Epub 2023 May 29. PMID: 37269620.

Sawicki GS, Lewis CL, and Ferris DP. It Pays to Have a Spring in Your Step. *Exerc Sport Sci Rev*. 2009 Jul;37(3):130-8. https://doi.org/10.1097/JES.0b013e31819c2df6. PMID: 19550204; PMCID: PMC2821187.

Shih Y, Chen YC, Lee YS, Chan MS, and Shiang TY. Walking Beyond Preferred Transition Speed Increases Muscle Activations With a Shift from Inverted Pendulum to Spring Mass Model in Lower Extremity. *Gait Posture*. 2016 May;46:5-10. https://doi.org/10.1016/j.gaitpost.2016.01.003. Epub 2016 Feb 12. PMID: 27131169.

Veronese N, Stubbs B, Volpato S, Zuliani G, Maggi S, Cesari M, Lipnicki DM, Smith L, Schofield P, Firth J, Vancampfort D, Koyanagi A, Pilotto A, and Cereda E. Association Between Gait Speed With Mortality, Cardiovascular Disease and Cancer: A

Systematic Review and Meta-Analysis of Prospective Cohort Studies. *J Am Med Dir Assoc*. 2018 Nov;19(11):981-988.e7. https://doi.org/10.1016/j.jamda.2018.06.007. Epub 2018 Jul 25. PMID: 30056008.

CHAPTER 6

Fradkin AJ, Zazryn TR, and Smoliga JM. Effects of Warming-Up on Physical Performance: A Systematic Review With Meta-Analysis. *J Strength Cond Res*. 2010 Jan;24(1):140-8. https://doi.org/10.1519/JSC.0b013e3181c643a0. PMID: 19996770.

McGowan CJ, Pyne DB, Thompson KG, and Rattray B. Warm-Up Strategies for Sport and Exercise: Mechanisms and Applications. *Sports Med*. 2015 Nov;45(11):1523-46. https://doi.org/10.1007/s40279-015-0376-x. PMID: 26400696.

Seeber GH, Wilhelm MP, Sizer PS Jr, Guthikonda A, Matthijs A, Matthijs OC, Lazovic D, Brismée JM, and Gilbert KK. The Tensile Behaviors of the Iliotibial Band: A Cadaveric Investigation. *Int J Sports Phys Ther*. 2020 May;15(3):451-459. PMID: 32566381; PMCID: PMC7296993.

Van Hooren B, and Peake JM. Do We Need a Cool-Down After Exercise? A Narrative Review of the Psychophysiological Effects and the Effects on Performance, Injuries and the Long-Term Adaptive Response. *Sports Med*. 2018 Jul;48(7):1575-1595. https://doi.org/10.1007/s40279-018-0916-2. PMID: 29663142; PMCID: PMC5999142.

CHAPTER 7

Atakan MM, Li Y, Koşar ŞN, Turnagöl HH, and Yan X. Evidence-Based Effects of High-Intensity Interval Training on Exercise Capacity and Health: A Review With Historical Perspective. *Int J Environ Res Public Health*. 2021 Jul 5;18(13):7201. https://doi.org/10.3390/ijerph18137201. PMID: 34281138; PMCID: PMC8294064.

Haggerty M, Dickin DC, Popp J, and Wang H. The Influence of Incline Walking on Joint Mechanics. *Gait Posture*. 2014 Apr;39(4):1017-21. https://doi.org/10.1016/j.gaitpost.2013.12.027. Epub 2014 Jan 8. PMID: 24472218.

Laukkanen JA, Voutilainen A, Kurl S, Araujo CGS, Jae SY, and Kunutsor SK. Handgrip Strength Is Inversely Associated With Fatal Cardiovascular and All-Cause Mortality Events. *Ann Med*. 2020 May-Jun;52(3-4):109-119. https://doi.org/10.1080/07853890.2020.1748220. Epub 2020 Apr 9. PMID: 32223654; PMCID: PMC7877981.

Masuki S, Morikawa M, and Nose H. Interval Walking Training Can Increase Physical Fitness in Middle-Aged and Older People. *Exerc Sport Sci Rev*. 2017 Jul;45(3):154-162. https://doi.org/10.1249/JES.0000000000000113. PMID: 28418999.

Mendes R, Sousa N, Themudo-Barata JL, and Reis VM. High-Intensity Interval Training Versus Moderate-Intensity Continuous Training in Middle-Aged and Older Patients With Type 2 Diabetes: A Randomized Controlled Crossover Trial of the Acute Effects of Treadmill Walking on Glycemic Control. *Int J Environ Res Public Health*. 2019 Oct 28: 16(21):4163. https://doi.org/10.3390/ijerph16214163.

Nakamura T, Kamiya K, Hamazaki N, Matsuzawa R, Nozaki K, Ichikawa T, Yamashita M, Maekawa E, Reed JL, Noda C, Meguro K, Yamaoka-Tojo M, Matsunaga A, and Ako J. Quadriceps Strength and Mortality in Older Patients With Heart Failure. *Can J Cardiol*. 2021 Mar;37(3):476-483. https://doi.org/10.1016/j.cjca.2020.06.019. Epub 2020 Jul 3. PMID: 32622879.

Newman AB, Kupelian V, Visser M, Simonsick EM, Goodpaster BH, Kritchevsky SB, Tylavsky FA, Rubin SM, and Harris TB. Strength, But Not Muscle Mass, Is Associated With Mortality in the Health, Aging and Body Composition Study Cohort. *J Gerontol A Biol Sci Med Sci*. 2006 Jan;61(1):72-7. https://doi.org/10.1093/gerona/61.1.72. PMID: 16456196.

Rijk JM, Roos PR, Deckx L, van den Akker M, and Buntinx F. Prognostic Value of Handgrip Strength in People Aged 60 Years and Older: A Systematic Review and Meta-Analysis. *Geriatr Gerontol Int*. 2016 Jan;16(1):5-20. https://doi.org/10.1111/ggi.12508. Epub 2015 May 28. PMID: 26016893.

Sen S, and Singh, AD. Influence of Carrying Loads on Ratings of Perceived Exertion and Heart Rate During Walking. *J Ergonomics*. 2016 6. 10.4172/2165-7556.1000176.

Wang HH, Tsai WC, Chang CY, Hung MH, Tu JH, Wu T, and Chen CH. Effect of Load Carriage Lifestyle on Kinematics and Kinetics of Gait. *Appl Bionics Biomech*. 2023 Feb 8;2023:8022635. https://doi.org/10.1155/2023/8022635. PMID: 36816755; PMCID: PMC9931482.

CHAPTER 8

Duñabeitia I, Arrieta H, Rodriguez-Larrad A, Gil J, Esain I, Gil SM, Irazusta J, and Bidaurrazaga-Letona I. Effects of Massage and Cold Water Immersion After an Exhaustive Run on Running Economy and Biomechanics: A Randomized Controlled Trial. *J Strength Cond Res*. 2022 Jan 1;36(1):149-155. https://doi.org/10.1519/JSC.0000000000003395. PMID: 31800477.

Dupuy O, Douzi W, Theurot D, Bosquet L, and Dugué B. An Evidence-Based Approach for Choosing Post-Exercise Recovery Techniques to Reduce Markers of Muscle Damage, Soreness, Fatigue, and Inflammation: A Systematic Review With Meta-Analysis. *Front Physiol*. 2018 Apr 26;9:403. https://doi.org/10.3389/fphys.2018.00403. PMID: 29755363; PMCID: PMC5932411.

Field T, Hernandez-Reif M, Diego M, Schanberg S, and Kuhn C. Cortisol Decreases and Serotonin and Dopamine Increase Following Massage Therapy. Int J Neurosci. 2005 Oct;115(10):1397-413. https://doi.org/10.1080/00207450590956459. PMID: 16162447.

Laffaye G, Da Silva DT, and Delafontaine A. Self-Myofascial Release Effect With Foam Rolling on Recovery After High-Intensity Interval Training. *Front Physiol*. 2019 Oct 16;10:1287. https://doi.org/10.3389/fphys.2019.01287. PMID: 31681002; PMCID: PMC6805773.

Şahin N, Karahan AY, and Albayrak İ. Effectiveness of Physical Therapy and Exercise on Pain and Functional Status in Patients With Chronic Low Back Pain: A Randomized-Controlled Trial. *Turk J Phys Med Rehabil*. 2017 Aug 9;64(1):52-58. https://doi.org/10.5606/tftrd.2018.1238. PMID: 31453489; PMCID: PMC6709610.

Vora M, Curry E, Chipman A, Matzkin E, and Li X. Patellofemoral Pain Syndrome in Female Athletes: A Review of Diagnoses, Etiology and Treatment Options. *Orthop Rev (Pavia)*. 2018 Feb 20;9(4):7281. https://doi.org/10.4081/or.2017.7281. PMID: 29564075; PMCID: PMC5850065.

CHAPTER 9

Beck BR, Daly RM, Singh MA, and Taaffe DR. Exercise and Sports Science Australia (ESSA) Position Statement on Exercise Prescription for the Prevention and Management of Osteoporosis. *J Sci Med Sport*. 2017 May;20(5):438-445. https://doi.org/10.1016/j.jsams.2016.10.001. Epub 2016 Oct 31. PMID: 27840033.

Canadian Society for Exercise Physiology. 2021. Canadian 24-Hour Movement Guidelines for Adults Aged 18-64 Years: An Integration of Physical Activity, Sedentary Behaviour, and Sleep. https://csepguidelines.ca/guidelines/adults-18-64/.

Cooper, KH. 1999. *Regaining the Power of Youth at Any Age*. Thomas Nelson, 1999.

European Union. 2008. EU Physical Activity Guidelines: Recommended Policy Actions in Support of Health-Enhancing Physical Activity. https://ec.europa.eu/assets/eac/sport/library/policy_documents/eu-physical-activity-guidelines-2008_en.pdf.

Gioftsidou A, Ispirlidis I, Pafis G, Malliou P, Bikos C, and Godolias G. Isokinetic Strength Training Program for Muscular Imbalances in Professional Soccer Players. *Sport Sci Health*. 2008;2:101-105. https://doi.org/10.1007/s11332-008-0047-5.

Gordon BR, McDowell CP, Lyons M, and Herring MP. The Effects of Resistance Exercise Training on Anxiety: A Meta-Analysis and Meta-Regression Analysis of Randomized Controlled Trials. *Sports Med*. 2017 Dec;47(12):2521-2532. https://doi.org/10.1007/s40279-017-0769-0. PMID: 28819746.

Kekäläinen T, Kokko K, Sipilä S, and Walker S. Effects of a 9-Month Resistance Training Intervention on Quality of Life, Sense of Coherence, and Depressive Symptoms in Older Adults: Randomized Controlled Trial. *Qual Life Res*. 2018 Feb;27(2):455-465. https://doi.org/10.1007/s11136-017-1733-z. Epub 2017 Nov 9. PMID: 29124498; PMCID: PMC5846971.

Kobayashi Y, Long J, Dan S, Johannsen NM, Talamoa R, Raghuram S, Chung S, Kent K, Basina M, Lamendola C, Haddad F, Leonard MB, Church TS, and Palaniappan L. Strength Training Is More Effective Than Aerobic Exercise for Improving Glycaemic Control and Body Composition in People With Normal-Weight Type 2 Diabetes: A Randomised Controlled Trial. *Diabetologia*. 2023 Oct;66(10):1897-1907. https://doi.org/10.1007/s00125-023-05958-9. Epub 2023 Jul 26. Erratum in: Diabetologia. 2024 Apr 30; PMID: 37493759; PMCID: PMC10527535.

Lauersen JB, Andersen TE, and Andersen LB. Strength Training as Superior, Dose Dependent, and Safe Prevention of Acute and Overuse Sports Injuries: A Systematic Review, Qualitative Analysis and Meta-Analysis. *Br J Sports Med*. 2018 Dec;52(24):1557-1563. https://doi.org/10.1136/bjsports-2018-099078. Epub 2018 Aug 21. PMID: 30131332.

Lee J, Kim D, and Kim C. Resistance Training for Glycemic Control, Muscular Strength, and Lean Body Mass in Old Type 2 Diabetic Patients: A Meta-Analysis. *Diabetes Ther*. 2017 Jun;8(3):459-473. https://doi.org/10.1007/s13300-017-0258-3. Epub 2017 Apr 5. PMID: 28382531; PMCID: PMC5446383.

MacDonald HV, Johnson BT, Huedo-Medina TB, Livingston J, Forsyth KC, Kraemer WJ, Farinatti PT, and Pescatello LS. Dynamic Resistance Training as Stand-Alone Antihypertensive Lifestyle Therapy: A Meta-Analysis. J Am Heart Assoc. 2016 Sep 28;5(10):e003231. https://doi.org/10.1161/JAHA.116.003231. PMID: 27680663; PMCID: PMC5121472.

Maestroni L, Read P, Bishop C, Papadopoulos K, Suchomel TJ, Comfort P, and Turner A. The Benefits of Strength Training on Musculoskeletal System Health: Practical Applications for Interdisciplinary Care. *Sports Med*. 2020 Aug;50(8):1431-1450. https://doi.org/10.1007/s40279-020-01309-5. PMID: 32564299.

Momma H, Kawakami R, Honda T, and Sawada SS. Muscle-Strengthening Activities Are Associated With Lower Risk and Mortality in Major Non-Communicable Diseases: A Systematic Review and Meta-Analysis of Cohort Studies. *Br J Sports Med*. 2022 Jul;56(13):755-763.

Mosti MP, Carlsen T, Aas E, Hoff J, Stunes AK, and Syversen U. Maximal Strength Training Improves Bone Mineral Density and Neuromuscular Performance in Young Adult Women. *J Strength Cond Res*. 2014 Oct;28(10):2935-45. https://doi.org/10.1519/JSC.0000000000000493. PMID: 24736773.

National Center for Health Statistics. Physical Activity Among Adults Ages 18 and Older: United States, 2020, National Health Interview Survey. www.cdc.gov/nchs/fastats/exercise.htm.

Sherrington C, Fairhall NJ, Wallbank GK, Tiedemann A, Michaleff ZA, Howard K, Clemson L, Hopewell S, and Lamb SE. Exercise for Preventing Falls in Older People Living in the Community. *Cochrane Database Syst Rev*. 2019 Jan;1(1):CD012424. https://doi.org/10.1002/14651858.CD012424.pub2. PMID: 30703272; PMCID: PMC6360922.

Shiroma EJ, Cook NR, Manson JE, Moorthy MV, Buring JE, Rimm EB, and Lee IM. Strength Training and the Risk of Type 2 Diabetes and Cardiovascular Disease. *Med Sci Sports Exerc*. 2017 Jan;49(1):40-46. https://doi.org/10.1249/MSS.0000000000001063. PMID: 27580152; PMCID: PMC5161704.

Statistics Canada. 2021. Canadian Health Measures Survey: Activity Monitor Data, 2018-2019. https://www150.statcan.gc.ca/n1/daily-quotidien/210901/dq210901c-eng.htm.

Suchomel TJ, Nimphius S, Bellon CR, and Stone MH. The Importance of Muscular Strength: Training Considerations. *Sports Med*. 2018 Apr;48(4):765-785. https://doi.org/10.1007/s40279-018-0862-z. PMID: 29372481.

U.S. Department of Health and Human Services. Physical Activity Guidelines for Americans, 2018, 2nd ed. Washington, DC: U.S. Department of Health and Human Services. https://odphp.health.gov/sites/default/files/2019-09/Physical_Activity_Guidelines_2nd_edition.pdf.

Westcott WL. Resistance Training Is Medicine: Effects of Strength Training on Health. *Curr Sports Med Rep*. 2012 Jul-Aug;11(4):209-16. https://doi.org/10.1249/JSR.0b013e31825dabb8. PMID: 22777332.

Yarizadeh H, Eftekhar R, Anjom-Shoae J, Speakman JR, and Djafarian K. The Effect of Aerobic and Resistance Training and Combined Exercise Modalities on Subcutaneous Abdominal Fat: A Systematic Review and Meta-Analysis of Randomized Clinical Trials. *Adv Nutr*. 2021 Feb 1;12(1):179-196. https://doi.org/10.1093/advances/nmaa090. PMID: 32804997; PMCID: PMC7849939.

CHAPTER 10

Canadian Society for Exercise Physiology. Canadian 24-Hour Movement Guidelines for Adults Aged 18-64 Years: An Integration of Physical Activity, Sedentary Behaviour, and Sleep. 2021. https://csepguidelines.ca/guidelines/adults-18-64/.

Nieman DC, Henson DA, Austin MD, and Sha W. Upper Respiratory Tract Infection Is Reduced in Physically Fit and Active Adults. *Br J Sports Med*. 2011 Sep;45(12):987-92. https://doi.org/10.1136/bjsm.2010.077875. Epub 2010 Nov 1. PMID: 21041243.

Nygaard H, Tomten SE, and Høstmark AT. Slow Postmeal Walking Reduces Postprandial Glycemia in Middle-Aged Women. *Appl Physiol Nutr Metab*. 2009 Dec;34(6):1087-92. https://doi.org/10.1139/H09-110. PMID: 20029518.

U.S. Department of Health and Human Services. Physical Activity Guidelines for Americans, 2018, 2nd ed. Washington, DC: U.S. Department of Health and Human Services. https://odphp.health.gov/sites/default/files/2019-09/Physical_Activity_Guidelines_2nd_edition.pdf.

CHAPTER 11

Adhikari, S, and Patil, PP. Effect of Uphill, Level, and Downhill Walking on Cardiovascular Parameters Among Young Adults. *Indian Journal of Health Sciences and Biomedical Research (KLEU)* 11(2): 121-124, May–Aug 2018. https://doi.org/10.4103/kleuhsj.kleuhsj_79_17.

Atakan, MM, Li Y, Koşar ŞN, Turnagöl HH, and Yan X. Evidence-Based Effects of High-Intensity Interval Training on Exercise Capacity and Health: A Review With Historical Perspective. *Int J Environ Res Public Health*. 2021 Jul 5;18(13):7201. https://doi.org/10.3390/ijerph18137201. PMID: 34281138; PMCID: PMC8294064.

Connolly, DA. The Energy Expenditure of Snowshoeing in Packed vs. Unpacked Snow at Low-Level Walking Speeds. *J Strength Cond Res*. 2002 Nov;16(4):606-10. PMID: 12423193.

Masood, Z, and Kobsar, D. The Effects of Incline Walking on Gait Asymmetry and Impact Accelerations in Patients With Knee Osteoarthritis. *Journal of Osteoarthritis and Cartilage* 29, supplement 1 (April 2021): S76-77.

ABOUT THE AUTHOR

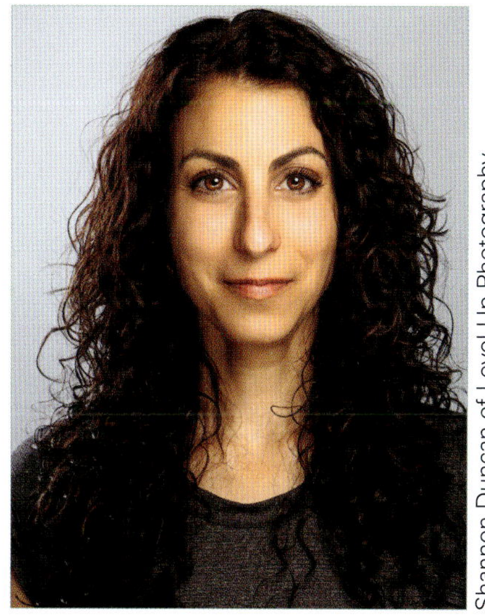

Shannon Duncan of Level Up Photography

Sarah Zahab is a Registered Kinesiologist, a member of the College of Kinesiologists of Ontario, a clinical exercise physiologist, and an award-winning fitness presenter with over 25 years of full-time fitness industry experience. She studied human kinetics at the University of Ottawa and graduated with honors with a bachelor of science degree.

A former international fitness competitor, Zahab proudly represented Canada at the Ms. Fitness World competition four times. She has been a nationally ranked race walker and is the 2012 and 2014 winner of the Ontario race walk championships (5,000 m) as well as the 2016 winner of the Canadian indoor national championship (3,000 m).

Zahab is the owner of Continuum Fitness and Movement Performance, a multidisciplinary clinic in Ottawa helping individuals move forward along their health continuum. She can be reached on social media at @continuumfit.

She enjoys spending time with her husband, John, and two daughters, and daily walks with her chocolate lab, Moka.

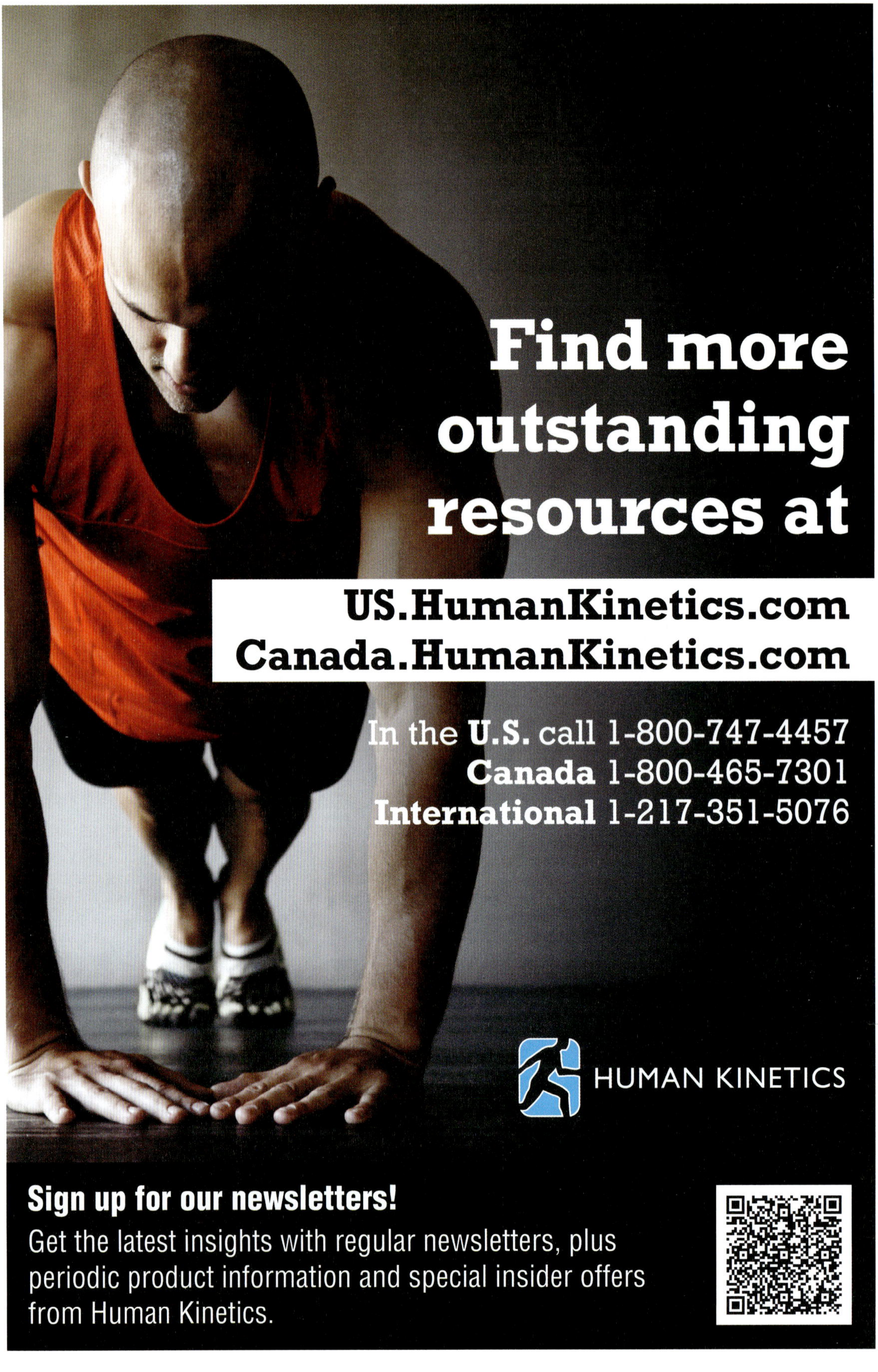